Susan Scott
MSc, FCIPD, FISMA, MABP, MBANT, Dip ION

LIFE FORCE

The revolutionary 7-step plan for optimum energy

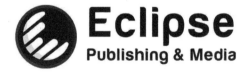

LIFE FORCE

The revolutionary 7-step plan for optimum energy

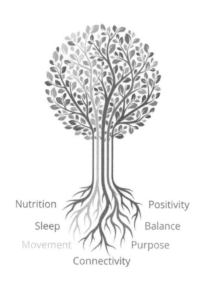

By Susan Scott MSc FCIPD FISMA MABP MBANT

The Energy Aunt

© 2019 Susan Scott

First published in Great Britain in 2019 by
Eclipse Publishing & Media Ltd, 22 Hillcrest, Tunbridge Wells, Kent, TN4 0AJ
www.epmbooks.co.uk

All rights reserved. No part of this publication may be reproduced, stored in a retrieval system, or transmitted, in any form or by any means, electronic, mechanical, photocopying, recording or otherwise, without the prior written permission of the publisher. Reprographic reproduction is permitted in accordance with the terms and licences issued by the Copyright Licensing Agency.

Disclaimer

The author and publisher believe that the sources of information upon which this book is based are reliable and have made every effort to ensure the accuracy of the text. However, neither the publisher nor the author can accept any legal responsibility whatsoever for consequences that may arise from errors or omissions, or from any opinion or advice given.

This book is intended as general information only. It is not intended to replace professional medical advice, nor should it be used to diagnose or treat any health condition. For diagnosis or treatment of any medical problem, consult your own qualified medical practitioner. The publisher and author disclaim any liability arising directly or indirectly from the use of this book and are not responsible for any specific health needs that may require medical supervision and are not liable for any damages or negative consequences from any treatment, action, application or preparation, to any person reading or following the information in this book.

ISBN 978-1-912839-02-5 (paperback)
ISBN 978-1-912839-52-0 (ebook)

Cover design by Aimee Coveney
Copy-edited by Graham Hughes
Text design by Daisy Editorial

Illustrations: tree illustration by Nata-Art/Shutterstock; sympathetic and parasympathetic system illustrations by Alila Medical Media/Shutterstock; edit and bulb icons by IYIKON from the Noun Project; notebook page image by FORGEM at iStock

Printed in Great Britain by Short Run Press Ltd.
Distributed by UK: Roundhouse Group/Orca
                US: SCB Distributors

Contents

To Helen Lewis, for making it happen

Endorsements

"I read this book with an increasing and alarming sense of recognition: Yep, did that. Yep, do that a lot. Yep, that's me. All in the bad, energy-sapping sense. If like me you have huge work–life balance challenges, especially with business travel, you should definitely read this. We all need to know more about managing energy and fatigue. I learned a lot that I didn't know about why energy's so vital and where it comes from. And also about what to do and what not to do. I found I did a lot of the latter! Susan Scott's book is so good because she looks both at the mind and body sides of energy. There aren't many authors who have genuine expertise and authority in both areas. If you implement what Susan recommends, even only parts of it, it will transform how you feel most of the time. I'm going to and I'm sure it will make a big difference."

– Dr Alan Bradshaw, Business Psychologist, Work–life Solutions Ltd

"Susan is a truly fabulous person. Having worked with her as a Resilience Trainer she has subsequently supported me with my personal nutrition in order to increase my own energy levels and wellbeing. When we met I was very low, exhausted and generally unhappy with my physical and mental health. Susan's expertise, combined with her high level of compassion and empathy, has truly helped me to understand more about nutrition and have access to a wide range of strategies and techniques to further support my development and recovery and improve my life. I would highly recommend her and am so happy to see all of this knowledge available in this book for more people to have access to."

– Ann Pemberton, Managing Director, Open Road Learning Ltd

"Anyone who's read either of Susan's previous books will know they are in for a treat. Not only are they packed with proven actions for you to take, but they are also written in a manner that makes the book personal to you – she is speaking only to you. There is much that will instantly resonate with you – about your level of energy generally, and about the experiences you may have felt at different times in your life. We all suffer from low energy levels at some time. And it's not surprising; the pace of life is frenetic; the need to maintain concentration is ever more challenging; the requirement to come to a rapid judgement and decision is ever present. Pausing for breath is now a luxury, whereas it should be a necessity, built in to the daily routine. Susan approaches the energy deficit challenge by providing each of you with a holistic and comprehensive approach to boosting energy. Like so many challenges, this one is best addressed from a complete person point of view, and not simply either nutrition or sport or something else, expecting it to have an impact on you as a whole. That doesn't work. Only a whole-person approach stands any chance of helping you adjust to the need to focus attention on YOU.

"This self-help book has seven steps. Follow them and you'll discover much more about yourself and what you should be doing to help yourself. The book provides tips – tips of icebergs, as beneath each tip is a whole science that has experimented in so many different ways – to produce a succinct and effective tip. Her best tip is 'be kind to yourself'. Beneath this tip is a huge foundation of psychological theories and principles that has demonstrated beyond argument that treating yourself (and others) with kindness plays to so many positive triggers that make you feel psychologically well – and, therefore, energised. You will discover information about your health you won't have even heard of; but take heart, it's all in the book to make you more aware of yourself, and what you need to do to boost your core energy and have a fantastic life."

– Dr Derek Mowbray, Chairman, The WellBeing and Performance Group, Independent Technical Expert to the European Commission on psychological wellbeing

"Ten years ago my life was turned upside down when I had an adverse reaction to an inoculation. I had to leave my job because of persistent fatigue and the symptoms and effects of IBS controlled my life every day. Then I was lucky enough to meet Susan and I knew that 'The Cavalry' had arrived. At last I had someone who had an explanation for what had happened to me; a plan to get my energy back and the knowledge to make it happen. In a nutshell, that is what this wonderful book will do for you. Susan's 7 steps to optimum energy will direct you and get you back on track. This book is a comprehensive cornucopia of everything you need to know in order to feel good and it will give you a clear understanding of how to overcome any hurdles to having great vitality."

– Isabel Sharma

"If your energy levels have taken a dive and you need to work on improving them, then 'Life Force' captures this beautifully using Susan's genuine 7-step plan. It helps you to understand where you are and recommends ways to get you motivated in order to get the most out of your life journey and to always feel good about yourself. I particularly enjoyed the connectivity chapter, which reinforced the importance of getting out and meeting new people. Taking part in a group exercise class provides a safe environment for escapism and allows you to let go with other like-minded people. Being stimulated in a room of happy people working out together helps you to stay buzzed for the rest of the day making you more powerful and enjoyable to be around."

– Kate Shaw, Award-winning fitness instructor, Surrey Dance Fitness, Winners Best Fitness Facility and Best Female Instructor, National Community Fitness Awards 2016

Introduction

Do *you* feel energised? What I mean is: do you spring out of bed in the morning, full of vitality and enthusiasm, and see through the day with passion and enthusiasm?

Or is it more like this – do you crawl out of bed and require copious amounts of coffee or sugary drinks to stand any chance of being able to focus and perform? Do you then just about manage to drag yourself through the day's activities, doing the minimum you can get away with as that's all you can do, while self-medicating along the way, taking whatever will give you a lift? At the end of the day, do you collapse into bed, drained and exhausted?

It sounds such a simple set of questions, and yet I bet if you're reading this book, your answer to the first question is "not very often" or even a resounding "no".

Being 'energised' means feeling wide awake, ready for whatever the day brings, having enough energy to do what you want, when you want. It's about feeling that every part of your body is functioning well and in harmony; that you have the physical and mental capability to perform to your best. It's a fabulous feeling!

Ask yourself: how often do you feel like that?

If your answer is "not enough" or "not often enough", then things need to change – and they can change. Life is far too precious to spend it feeling like every day should be a duvet day. Stop feeling tired all the time.

Why you need this book

Well, it's very simple – do you want to:

- enhance your energy, vitality and sustainability?
- fuel the energy-making powerhouses in your body?
- avoid energy slumps during the day?
- sleep better and wake revitalised?
- use energy to focus, concentrate and deliver to a higher standard?
- improve your mood and outlook on life?
- improve your resilience to manage your demanding life?
- be able to live life to the full?

Yes? Then this book is for you.

Only you can put things right. Life is no longer straightforward. Demands on your time and energy are increasing. Home, work, relationships and commitments all try to take a piece of you.

The pace of life is growing at a phenomenal rate. We now work longer hours and cut back on recreation and 'me' time. But if you're going to avoid burning out, you need to take action. You need to do all you can to keep your energy bank topped up. To be clear: you cannot afford not to.

This book is unique! It is not your usual diet or detox book that only tells you half the story so you feel better for a while then crash again. It will tell you all you need to know, physically, mentally and emotionally. From how to support your body's energy-making process to how to train your mind to generate energy as well. You might not need it all, but I can confidently say that there will be something here that will help you.

I am unique! I am exactly the right person to tell you how to get more energy. As a professional business psychologist and registered nutritional therapist, I will use my professionally guided, evidence-based mind *and* body approach to explain what you need to eat, drink and think in a way that heals your body and gives you the energy required to not only cope, but thrive.

What really brings my message alive, though, is that I've lived with low energy and I know just how ghastly it is. I know what it's like to think, "What's wrong with me? I can usually do this." I know what it's like to feel that I should be able to do something easily but that I just don't have the energy. It's frustrating, it's frightening and it's flippin' awful. When you're struggling with a lack of energy, it's hard to see a way out – but I did. Let me tell you more.

My story

I had always been a high-energy girl. Driven, hard-working and creative. Over the years I've had business success, including a very successful consulting career as a business psychologist which had me travelling the world. I ran a busy clinic for stressed-out executives and I've had the privilege of being chair of the stress industry's professional association, the International Stress Management Association. I always want to be 'doing'. But the reality has been that this has not always been possible, to the extent that I feared for my very life.

Health has always been my passion. I would put my interest in health as one of my top three core values. As a teenager I trotted off to a weekly yoga class (I've still no idea where this came from, as no one in my family did anything like this) and I even wanted to be a dietitian, but life got in the way.

The problem is, I started life with bundles of energy and felt everything was in my grasp with a bit of hard work, but, eighteen years ago, life changed all that. I felt utterly exhausted. Whereas I used to be able to work hard and play hard and recharge with a couple of early nights, suddenly I didn't even have the energy to play if I was going to function at my work. My doctor said there was nothing wrong with me – repeatedly over an eighteen-month period. I knew there was. Not only did I have no energy, but I ached all over, and the brain fog I was experiencing meant my memory was shot and I struggled to think straight. The morning's activities would wipe me out and I'd spend the afternoon curled up on the sofa – I couldn't even get up to get a glass of water. At the time I was studying for my psychology Master of Science degree. Things got so bad, I really began to think that I'd have to pull out.

On a return trip to my doctor, I happened to see his computer screen and noticed that my test results were showing I had an under-functioning thyroid. A fluke, he said. I was anaemic (I had that too). I persuaded him to refer me to an endocrinology consultant, who told me I was very ill and my life would never be the same again – not the best thing to hear when you've been a high-energy person. He was right. Having an autoimmune thyroid condition (Hashimoto's thyroiditis) is like walking an energy tightrope and so many factors can trigger a low-energy state. There's so much more to it than taking a small pill every day. I recovered well enough to function, but not to how I had been before.

Two years later, I began to live the dream I had had as a teenager and studied nutrition at the renowned Institute for Optimum Nutrition (ION). This was a professional must, because my coaching experience was telling me that you couldn't improve behaviour and wellbeing without considering both the mind and body.

I studied ION's three-year diploma and foundation science degree course. I loved it. Despite all the difficulties of studying and working full-time, as well as travelling with my work and being mum to two teenagers, I coped (just), and my energy improved. I even graduated with distinction.

Then a blip came another couple of years down the line. I was exhausted again, and tests showed my liver enzymes were elevated – a virus from my travels, said the consultant. I recovered. Then a few years ago the symptoms started again, despite my taking my medication, watching my diet and taking some supplements. This time the aches in my soft tissue were back, and I got to the stage where I feared for my future mobility.

A friend from my ION days who was studying for a PhD referred me onto a biochemistry research programme, and very quickly it was discovered that I had toxic metal poisoning: nickel from my stainless-steel saucepans – can you believe it? The programme I undertook to clear it was ghastly, but one day I woke up and thought "welcome back" – my real self had returned.

When I reflect on these years, I notice that every time I've had an 'episode' I've been very stressed, in fact struggling with adrenal fatigue and on the verge of burnout. My experiences and my mind/body studies as a business psychologist and nutritionist have helped me enormously. I want to share this knowledge and reassure others that you can recover your energy. You can change your mindset and add practices to your life to make you the person you truly are.

2017 was a big year for me... and rather stressful for several reasons. I wrote and published two books around the theme of career performance, stress and burnout. Both books went to #1 on Amazon!

One book is tough to do and two was probably madness, but my energy and enthusiasm to share my message pushed me to do it. I ended the year with an amazing trip to Asia. The diet and spiritual learning were incredible, but the pollution in the cities triggered a relapse in my autoimmune thyroid condition. I came home chronically fatigued and coughing. I now accept that these blips will occur from time to time, but I'm reassured that I have the tools and techniques to get myself back to firing on all cylinders – and this is the best feeling.

Why managing your energy is so important

As Mark Twain said, "And what is a man without energy? Nothing – nothing at all." I know just how right he was.

Everything you do, every natural and intentional function you perform, draws on your energy. You need physical energy to move and function, you need mental energy to direct your thinking and learn, and you need emotional energy for relationships.

It's not so very different to your smartphone. How frustrated and irritated do you feel when it runs out of battery power? I would suggest you would be pretty high on the frustrated and irritated scale. To prevent this from happening, you diligently plug your phone in each evening to recharge the battery, so you can feel safe and confident that it will be fired up and fully functioning to perform whatever you demand of it the next day. Well, your body is no different. It works in exactly the same way – it uses energy, and that energy needs replenishing. If you don't recharge your body's batteries, then you will eventually stop functioning.

You cannot expect your body to perform well regardless of what you demand from it, and you certainly should not take your energy for granted. Energy is the foundation stone of your health and wellbeing. It fuels your productivity and rewards you with the riches you seek. It is life! And there's no way you can 'have it all', or anywhere close, without energy!

Energy is personal to you. Only you can do what is required to renew it, and it is your choice as to what action you take. You need to be prepared to take over the management of your energy. No one can do it for you. There is no magic pill – and if you think you've found one, the effects will only be temporary, and I dread to think what damage will be done.

Optimising your personal energy will take commitment and practice. Yes, you'll have to fit this in around all the other parts of your life you're also managing – such as relationships, children, finances and time – but if you're really honest with yourself, you know you'll stand little chance of success in managing all these other demands without energy. The time spent optimising your energy is an investment in you and a great life.

Why read this book?

Generating and maintaining high levels of energy should be a way of life that *you* do for yourself for the extent of your life. It should not be like making a New Year's resolution to go to the gym but giving up by the third week in January and going back to the way you were. You need to develop this as a lifelong practice, and my mission is to help you.

This book is a 'how-to' book, setting you off on your own journey of discovery of how you can successfully optimise your personal energy naturally and permanently. This type of sustainable energy comes from small adjustments to your diet, lifestyle and thinking. It uses my twin-track *mind and body* approach to look at all aspects of the real 'you'. It's the only way to ensure sustainable success which allows you to live the life you want.

Your energy is totally unique to you. I want to help you to understand what it takes to operate at your best. This book will tell you all you need to know. It is packed with descriptions, theory, a bit of science, and detailed explanations of where energy actually comes from and why it is important to manage it.

There are questionnaires and activities to complete, which will raise your personal awareness of the extent and limits of your energy and help you decide where you should focus your attention to achieve success. Each chapter explains a variety of techniques that have the potential to change your life if you practise them. And finally, real-life stories from my clinic and coaching practice will reassure you that you're not alone on this journey, that we all have challenges, but big gains can be made with a few small changes.

The good news is that you *can* live a life feeling full of energy. It just takes some changes to your diet and lifestyle and adding some simple yet effective practices into your daily routine to feel energised, motivated and engaged. By applying the steps in this book, you'll have a sharp mind and, above all, will be resilient enough to deal with the demands life places on you.

How to use this book

My book will introduce you to my **7 Steps to Optimum Energy** programme. It is a programme that covers your mind and body and all the components of the way you function as a person. Each step is an element in your life that has the potential to feed or zap your energy.

Step 1: Nutrition. This is the most basic requirement. Virtually every cell in your body contains little energy factories called *mitochondria* which primarily use blood glucose and a variety of nutrients to generate energy. Unless you are well nourished, nothing else will be able to optimise your energy.

Step 2: Sleep. You cannot function without sleep. You have evolved to use this time to restore, repair and recover from the strains of your time awake. You need good-quality sleep in sufficient quantity. If sleep is compromised, so is your energy.

Step 3: Movement. This is a vital component of the energy production process. Exercise increases oxygen to your cells and clears the waste product carbon dioxide from them.

Step 4: Connectivity. People need people. We're social animals and get so much of our energy from connecting with other people. Connecting with others makes you happy and engaged and can help you to switch off from the internal chatter that's exacerbating the stress you feel.

Step 5: Purpose. Purpose is your inner self, your spirit, the very energy that drives you. Knowing what's important to you, following your direction in life and living that dream feeds your sense of meaning and generates energy.

Step 6: Balance. Life can be stressful. Your body's mechanism for managing these challenges is to go into 'fight or flight' mode and release two hormones: adrenalin and cortisol. If you are leading a fast-paced, highly demanding life, you could be stuck in an 'always-on', high-stress-hormone state, and this will put huge demands on your energy.

Step 7: Positivity. Positivity is about the positive emotions that energise and motivate you. As part of your survival mechanism, you will be on alert for danger; this stimulates negative thinking pathways in your brain, which in turn lowers mood. Positivity creates chemicals in your brain that improve your outlook and energise you.

Within each step are seven 'energy-boosting' ways to improve your performance. Seven steps, each with seven ways, gives you forty-nine powerful tips that have the potential to change your life.

I've added one more to make it fifty! This fiftieth tip is the most powerful of all:

It's 'Be kind to yourself'.

Remember what I said earlier. If you want to boost your energy, then you need to put yourself at the heart of it. Getting to the stage where you need to read my book may well mean everyone and everything has come before you. This is your time and your territory. You owe it to yourself.

Work your way through the book. I will introduce to you what energy means and the factors in your life that have the potential to zap your energy from you. The purpose of this is to raise your awareness and prepare you for the programme.

You will then be introduced to the **7 Steps to Optimum Energy**. Each step is presented in its own chapter, and each chapter contains an explanation of the science behind the element and why this step has a place in energy production and maintenance – plus how this step has the potential to boost your energy. Seven ways will be suggested that will start you on your journey to optimising your personal energy. These are the seven most powerful practices that I have recognised in people, when working with them, that boost their energy.

At the start of each chapter you will be presented with questions that ask you how you feel and perform. Read them carefully and answer them honestly. If your answer to any of these questions is "Yes", then creating healthy rituals and new lifestyle habits is a must.

Towards the end of the chapter, there will be some written activities for you to complete. These will help you to identify the extent to which this element requires your attention. It will finish with an opportunity for you to reflect on what you have learned when reading this chapter, and which of the seven ways suggested you will practise to achieve that much-needed boost to your energy. You do not have to do all seven. Some you may already be doing; others may seem untenable to you at this time. Choose what will be the simplest for you to practise that gives you the best results.

Work your way through the book and read it with an open mind. It may become evident to you that some of the elements are functioning well – you may sleep well or be very active. This means you have already taken that step to optimise your energy. That is really good news. Still complete the reflection exercise, though, to explain why; and if there is anything else you can do, record it here.

Chapter 12 will allow you to capture the reflections you have made throughout the book, and the changes you can make to your diet and lifestyle that will boost your energy. When you review this chapter, be mindful that you cannot do it all. Firstly, you may be too exhausted; secondly, you may not have the capacity and time to do everything; and thirdly, the more you do, the less likely you are to continue. It will be much more beneficial if you start gently.

Following this programme will give you ways to improve your energy, and it will be easier than you might think. By making some simple changes in your daily life, you will soon understand how the world actually can be your oyster!

PART 1

Energy

CHAPTER 1

What is energy?

◊ Are you flagging as soon as you get up in the morning?

◊ Do you experience an afternoon slump in energy that makes it hard for you to focus and remain cheerful?

◊ Do you wonder just how you will get the energy together to meet the next deadline?

◊ Do you ever wonder if it's possible to feel bright and full of energy again?

◊ Does your brain feel foggy and do you have trouble concentrating?

◊ Are you exhausted and run ragged by your working life?

◊ Do you feel that you regularly ping-pong between wired and tired?

◊ Are you ready to stop that feeling of 'running on empty'?

If you've answered "Yes" to any of these questions, then you've purchased the right book!

Energy is your vitality and capacity to function and live your life. It's the very fuel in your tank that drives your motivation and capability to bring your skills to life and achieve what you want to achieve, from day-to-day functioning to achieving your goals and ambitions. It's your very essence of living.

Energy has an impact on you physically and mentally. It affects how well your body functions, so it therefore affects your health, as well as your thoughts, emotions, moods and behaviour. When you have an abundance of energy you feel alive, engaged, confident, joyful and creative. You're focused and alert; you can think clearly and decisively, and access memories with ease. You're thriving, not just surviving, and feel that you have the capacity to take on anything life throws at you.

However, when your energy is depleted, you're likely to feel unwell, down in the dumps, hopeless and overwhelmed by all you need to do. You struggle to function and achieve anything. Your capacity to cope has left you, and along with that, your resilience.

It's energy that helps you get more done, more easily and to a better standard. All the planning and preparation in the world counts for nothing if you haven't got the get-up-and-go to actually do it.

Life has changed in the last few years, and the way we live our lives now means that we struggle to maintain our energy. Life has become about being 'always-on', 'always-doing' and always striving for the 'must-haves', with little time allocated for reflection and recovery. Whereas we used to talk about work–life balance, where life at work ended and home life began, now they both blend into one. Digital technology, which blurs the lines between work and home, has put paid to that.

The reality, though, is that our full-on, always-doing lives leave us struggling to perform at our best 100 per cent of the time. I hear it all the time: "I wish I had more energy." It's almost becoming normal to feel tired all the time; many of us wouldn't know how it feels to be any other way. It's so prevalent in modern society that doctors even have a word for it: TATT or 'tired-all-the-time'.

Managing a demanding job and squeezing home life in around it does require a never-ending supply of energy to cope and perform well. This means that it's no longer just about managing your time (a big ask right now with the ever-increasing challenges, demands and interruptions) – you now need to manage your energy too.

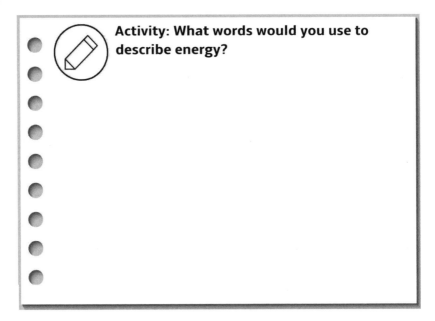

Activity: What words would you use to describe energy?

Part

1

Where does energy come from?

Every process in your body, from what you think to what you do, requires energy. It's what has you awake, standing up and functioning or, more to the point, alive. This type of energy, the fuel of life, is called *metabolic energy*.

Your body is made up of a variety of cells. Examples include muscle, nerve, heart, liver and blood cells. Every cell in your body, except for blood cells, metabolises glucose and oxygen, using specific processes to create energy.

In the same way that a car has an engine, your cells have one or more engines within them to give you the power to make you function. These engines, mitochondria, are tiny bean-shaped organelles. The number of mitochondria within the cell depends on its function and how much energy is required. It probably will come as no surprise that nerve, heart and muscle cells contain the most.

Mitochondria generate *adenosine triphosphate* (ATP) as fuel for the cell to do the job it is assigned to do. They do this by the oxidation of glucose into ATP, carbon dioxide and water. Glucose from carbohydrate is the most efficient food, but the body can convert protein and fat in the absence of glucose. The whole process requires two coordinated biochemical processes. The first to take place is the *citric acid cycle*, also known as the *tricarboxylic acid cycle* or *Krebs cycle*; this is then followed by the *electron transport chain*. About thirty molecules of ATP are produced per molecule of glucose. Both of these biochemical processes require certain nutrients to drive the chain of reaction. This is the reason why food is life, and why a balanced diet is so important. It's all very well having enough glucose, but if you don't have the nutrients to operate the biochemical processes, you won't generate energy and will instead just store the glucose as fat.

As I'm sure you can imagine, the human body has a high demand for ATP. It is made and used with great ferocity and speed, which is why some cells, such as the liver and heart, can hold up to 2000 mitochondria. Very little is kept in reserve. To make sure the process is as efficient as possible, unused ATP is being constantly recycled.

Part 1

Activities to identify what you know about your energy

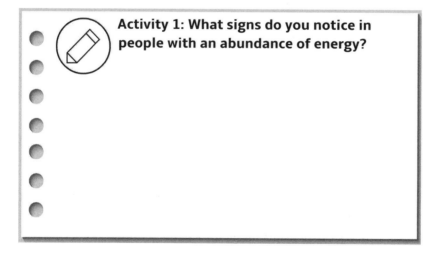

Activity 1: What signs do you notice in people with an abundance of energy?

Activity 2: How bright is your light?

How would you judge your current energy levels? What is the strength of your light bulb? Look at the statements and questions below and place a tick in the relevant column depending on whether always (100W), mostly (60W), sometimes (40W) or never (Bulb Blown).

	100W	60W	40W	Bulb Blown
I feel a vitality for life				
My energy remains good throughout all aspects of my life				
I wake in the morning and feel recharged				
I sustain my energy levels well throughout the day at work				
I sustain my energy levels well throughout the day when not at work				
I have the energy and enthusiasm to embrace whatever comes my way				
I have the energy and enthusiasm to give people the time they would like				
I come home from work with enthusiasm for my family, some exercise, or my hobby				
I feel calm, relaxed and ready to retire to bed at a similar time each evening				
Score				

Part 1

Look at the chart and take note of where you have scored the most.

If you have scored mostly '100W', your light bulb is shining brightly and you are brimming with energy and vitality.

If you have scored mostly '60W', you are still giving off sufficient brightness and have the energy to perform. There may still be changes you can make to your diet and lifestyle to brighten your light bulb further.

If you have scored mostly '40W', your bulb is dim and emitting very little light to help you function. You may struggle with fluctuating energy levels, so use this book to identify which aspects of your diet and lifestyle require improving and how you can incorporate healthy rituals into your everyday life.

If you scored mostly 'Bulb Blown', you may well be burnt out physically and mentally and be emotionally exhausted. This book will help you, but you also need to visit a specialist to help you recover.

Activity 3: Your life force

What feeds your energy? Think about examples as you're doing this.

- Physically – your body's physical health, such as the digestive, endocrine and nervous systems
- Mentally – your ability to focus, concentrate, remember and problem-solve
- Emotionally – your mood, feelings, confidence and resilience
- Socially – your relationships
- Spiritually – your meaning, purpose, passion and drive for life

Part 1

Energy elements	What feeds your energy
Physically	
Mentally	
Emotionally	
Socially	
Spiritually	

Your reflections

What has resonated with you while reading about energy?

- What have you learned about yourself?
- What have you learned about the state of your energy?
- What do you need to start doing that you have not done before?
- What other thoughts do you have?

CHAPTER 2

The energy zappers

I would hedge a bet that the very reason you're reading this book is because you're struggling with low energy and you're at a loss as to how to boost it.

We've learned that energy, our very basic life fuel, is produced in the mitochondria. These tiny powerhouses, like the engine in your car, are designed to run well and efficiently. However, this doesn't always happen, and if you are feeling uncharacteristically fatigued, there's every chance the function of your mitochondria has been compromised.

Fatigue is characterised by a lack of engagement, focus and motivation. This can be accompanied by tiredness, weakness, sleepiness, despondency or low mood. Fatigue can differ in severity. Mild fatigue is symptomatic of a feeling of tiredness, which can be corrected by a few early nights or taking some time out with a holiday. Moderate to severe fatigue is something quite different and will typically be the result of an impairment in the energy processing system. It could be a lack of stamina or endurance, and in extreme cases even the simplest tasks become difficult to perform and require a period of recovery before there is any chance of further activity.

Low metabolic energy is miserable. The only way to improve your energy to a healthy level is to identify the underlying cause and put practices or support in place to correct the issue. The factors that can impair mitochondrial function are:

- nutritional deficiencies
- malfunction of the thyroid or pancreatic glands
- chronic stress and adrenal exhaustion

Nutritional deficiencies

Is this you?
- You still feel bloated thirty minutes after eating
- You burp a lot thirty minutes after eating
- You have undigested food in your stools
- You suffer from heartburn, indigestion
- You have bad breath
- You cannot taste your food
- Cuts and grazes are slow to heal
- Your fingernails peel or break easily
- You have iron deficiency anaemia and supplementation is not improving the situation sufficiently

Yes? Then you may have a nutritional deficiency. There are a number of reasons for a deficiency in the key nutrients required for the energy production process.

» A lack of variety

A lack of variety in the diet is the primary cause of low energy. People do not eat enough food and have enough variety to provide the spread of nutrients required for the biochemical processes.

An intake of primarily processed foods will lack nutrients because they have been bleached or processed out. Vegans will miss out on vitamin B12, one of the most important nutrients for energy, because this is only found in animal products. The big fad for losing weight by following a ketogenic or paleo diet means carbohydrates are restricted. Fruit and vegetables are vitamin- and mineral-rich carbohydrates.

However, optimising nutrients is not always as straightforward as just eating a varied diet. That is, a diet balanced with a rainbow of different fruits and vegetables, and other nutritious foods such as nuts and seeds, meat and fish.

Nutritional deficiencies may also arise from how well you digest your food and how well you absorb the nutrients from your gut into your blood steam.

» Low stomach acid

Digestion begins in the stomach, where hydrochloric acid begins the process of breaking down protein, releasing minerals from foods and facilitating the absorption of vitamin B12. It also triggers other digestive enzymes, such as pancreatic enzymes, which digest food in the small intestines.

When the amount of stomach acid produced is low (*hypochlorhydria*), the process of breaking down food does not get off to a good start. The breakdown of food allows for the release of vitamins, minerals, amino acids and fatty acids ready for absorption into the bloodstream. If you feel bloated and gassy thirty minutes after eating, or notice undigested food in your stools, this could be the cause.

Stomach acid is also required to trigger the opening of the *pyloric valve*, a valve that connects the stomach to the top of the small intestine. A failure to trigger this leaves your food fermenting in your stomach and gas is created.

The causes of hypochlorhydria are many, but in my experience the main one is stress. Stressful events trigger the 'fight or flight' stress response. When you're trying to survive the threat of being eaten by a sabretooth tiger, the last thing you have time for is to grab a sandwich. One of the actions of the stress hormone cortisol is to slow digestion and peristalsis in the digestive tract. When this happens, you don't

Part
1

break your food down sufficiently for absorption. It can be made all the worse by not taking time out to eat. Grabbing a bite to eat and gobbling it down while sitting at your desk doing your emails could be the reason.

» Nutrient robbers

Eating well, by which I mean consuming a rich and varied diet, is important. You are what you eat! However, there may be aspects of your diet or lifestyle that are undoing some of the benefits you may think you're getting from your diet. What you eat can also be your nutrient undoing. I call these the *vitamin robbers*. Vitamin robbers either inhibit nutrient absorption or create an increased demand for nutrients, reducing the amount available for the energy production process.

Lifestyle factors such as tobacco smoking and alcohol reduce the absorption of vitamin C and increase your body's demand for it once absorbed, because vitamin C is a vital antioxidant. You could need as much as four times the intake to achieve the blood nutrient levels a non-smoker or teetotaller does. Certain drugs such as painkillers can have the same effect.

Pesticides, plastics and chemicals play havoc on the gut, impairing absorption. Drinking water straight from the tap contains hormone and plastic residues. Always filter your water. Eating organic isn't always possible, so the very minimum you should do is wash fruit and vegetables well when you've bought them and before you store them away or refrigerate them. I love grapes and they're high in nutrients, but if you could see the pollution in the San Fernando Valley in California where grapes are grown, you'd be shocked. Fruit is heavily sprayed with pesticides. I never eat an apple without washing it first! Yes, and I also peel carrots to minimise pesticide contamination. I use a plumbed-in water filter, and a new cartridge arrives every six months. Much better than worktop varieties which you can forget to change.

Using cling film to cook or microwaving food in cheap plastic containers increases your chemical load. Only use 'non-PVC' cling film. Plastic water bottles are only for one use, so don't reuse them.

Industrial and motor pollution is also an antinutrient. I returned from a fabulous trip to India chronically fatigued. I know the motor pollution was the culprit. Living in a city or by a busy road increases your exposure. Even driving short distances which include queuing in traffic sends the levels of exhaust fumes you breathe sky-high. You're actually better walking!

Contact with heavy metals – which are minerals but with no biological function – can, amongst other things, inhibit the absorption of certain vital minerals by taking priority over them. If your diet is low in a certain mineral, the heavy metal will mimic it and be absorbed. Lead takes priority over iron, calcium and copper, putting anyone in this situation at risk of iron, copper and calcium deficiency; and nickel will be absorbed if zinc is missing in the diet. Once a heavy metal is in the cell, it has the potential to weaken the energy production cycle by blocking enzyme binding sites, or by altering the antioxidant systems which clean the cell up from all the 'combustion' activity that takes place. Examples of heavy metals include lead, mercury, cadmium, aluminium and nickel. Lead is found in oil paint, and in some cosmetics and hair dyes. Mercury is found in amalgam fillings and certain fish (tuna, as a scavenging fish, is often contaminated). Cadmium is found in cigarettes, and in some fertilisers and industrial waste. Aluminium comes from foil, antiperspirants and cooking utensils, and nickel from stainless-steel cooking utensils and jewellery. The symptoms I've seen in clients with heavy metal poisoning frequently include fatigue. I even have personal experience, when I had nickel poisoning from my saucepans. I am very wary of toxic metals now. I try to avoid tuna fish. I would never encourage the use of amalgam fillings, and if I use aluminium foil for cooking, I avoid the use of citrus juice, such as lemon juice,

Part
1

as this frees the aluminium metal from the foil ready to be absorbed by the cooking food.

Your gut flora (*microbiome*) is like a little community inside your gut, working hard to keep you well. One of the roles of good bacteria is to manufacture B vitamins. B vitamins are essential for energy production. Too many courses of antibiotics and your microbiome will suffer.

Drugs can also be nutrient robbers. Painkillers, in particular aspirin, can irritate the gut, causing inflammation which upsets the absorption of nutrients. Statins inhibit the absorption of fat-soluble vitamins (A, D and E) and Coenzyme Q10 (CoQ10). CoQ10 is a key component of the energy manufacturing cycle. This is why many people experience pain in their muscles and soft tissues: they are struggling to manufacture energy. Thyroid hormone supplementation may inhibit the absorption of iron and calcium. This was a revelation to me when I struggled to understand why I experienced cramp so often. Hormone replacement therapy (HRT) and the contraceptive pill inhibit the absorption of zinc and the spectrum of B vitamins. Antidepressants and sleeping medication also affect zinc uptake, an essential component for energy. Antacids, diuretics and laxatives interfere with the absorption of a variety of nutrients. Quite a list, and why I always prefer to use food as medicine.

Food allergies can also produce inflammation in the gut. I am not a fan of cutting out dairy and gluten for 'health' reasons or because you're following a 'clean' diet. These two food groups are high in nutrients, including fibre, which feeds your microbiome. More on this in Chapter 4.

Here's something you might not have thought about. Is it best to eat your food raw or cook it? Surprisingly, raw is not always best. For many foods, cooking helps to break down tough fibrous walls and release nutrients. Tomatoes are an example of this. Cooked tomato contains more lycopene than uncooked.

There is so much more to this topic, it requires a whole book if I'm going to inform you better. For now, though, I want to start simply and raise your awareness so you think twice when you pour a glass of water from the tap or you eat unwashed fruit. Not only do these nutrient robbers reduce the vitamins and minerals available to you, but the residues get stored in your body, in fat deposits, muscles and soft tissues – in other words, in your cells – and this can affect your energy levels.

Conditions of the thyroid or pancreas

» Poor thyroid function

Is this you?
- Physically and mentally exhausted
- Dry or itchy or rough skin
- Cracked heels
- Hair which is dry and falling out
- Brittle, flaking nails
- Cold all the time
- Constipated
- Putting on weight
- Muscle, soft tissue and joint pain
- Lost the outer third of your eyebrows
- Brain fog – poor memory, concentration and focus
- Low mood
- Slow-to-heal cuts and grazes
- Sore throat or tightness at the front of your neck
- Heavy periods or infertility problems
- Yeast infections

Yes? These are symptoms of low metabolic energy that could be a sign of a thyroid gland disorder.

The thyroid gland is a butterfly-shaped gland located at the front of your neck, and is part of the endocrine system of glands that produce and secrete hormones to regulate the activity of cells or hormones.

The thyroid gland produces two hormones, primarily *thyroxine* (T4) and small amounts of *triiodothyronine* (T3). Thyroxine is the inactive form, which is converted in the liver to triiodothyronine, the biologically active form, which passes in your bloodstream to almost every cell in your body. It is required as part of the energy-making cycle to form ATP molecules, which then regulates the speed with which the cells undertake their function. If the manufacture of thyroxine is compromised, you will not be generating enough energy in the cell for it to fulfil its function. This is why an under-performing thyroid makes you feel so fatigued and sluggish. Its effects are felt in every part of the body because it affects every cell – and that's what we are: a mass of cells.

There are two reasons for an under-performing thyroid gland:

Nutritional deficiencies. The thyroid gland requires, amongst other nutrients, the amino acid L-tyrosine and iodine to manufacture the hormones, and the mineral selenium to convert T4 to T3. Vitamins D and A are required by the cell to receive T3. A nutrient supplementation plan will be required to address any deficiencies in any of these nutrients.

Hashimoto's thyroiditis. This is an autoimmune disease where the body's immune system attacks and gradually destroys the thyroid gland. This prevents the gland from releasing adequate levels of hormones. Blood tests performed by your doctor will determine whether antibodies are present and the levels of hormone released by the gland. Medication in the form of synthetic thyroid hormone is prescribed.

If you suspect your thyroid gland is under-performing, I would recommend you visit your doctor and request some thyroid-screening blood tests.

» Poor pancreatic function

Is this you?

- Frequently urinating; you even need to get up during the night
- Excessively thirsty
- Hungry all the time
- Losing weight
- Losing muscle bulk or definition
- Feeling tired and listless
- Blurred vision
- Having a tingling sensation or numbness in your hands or feet
- Finding it difficult to concentrate and focus
- Suffering with yeast infections (thrush)
- Slow-to-heal cuts and grazes?

Part

1

Yes? These are symptoms of low metabolic energy that could be a sign of diabetes, a pancreatic disorder.

Diabetes is a malfunction of the pancreas gland. The pancreas is a long gland sited deep in the abdomen near the stomach as part of the digestive system. It is also part of the endocrine system of glands, producing a number of important hormones.

The key pancreatic hormones relating to energy are insulin, which promotes the absorption of glucose from the bloodstream into the cells; glucagon, the opposite of insulin, which raises concentrations of glucose in the bloodstream; and pancreatic enzymes that assist in the breakdown of food and the absorption of nutrients in the small intestine.

I want to expand on insulin here, as this hormone has a big impact on mitochondrial functionality. Insulin allows your cells to use the glucose that has come from the carbohydrate food you have consumed. As soon as you eat and your digestive system breaks down carbohydrates into glucose and they are absorbed into the bloodstream, the beta cells in your pancreas will release insulin. Insulin attaches itself to the glucose and signals for the cell to absorb the glucose, provided that it needs it. I liken it to a key unlocking the door and allowing insulin in. If the cell has no room, glucose will be stored in the liver or as fat. The energy production cycle in the cell prioritises glucose over protein and fats for energy production; it produces more energy for less effort. If insulin is low – either because you have not been eating carbohydrates or because there is an impairment to the manufacture of insulin in the pancreas – then the body will process proteins and fats, the by-products of which are ammonia and ketones (hence the unpleasant breath and body odour from people on high-protein diets).

Pancreatic dysfunction can be a consequence of:

Consuming a diet high in processed carbohydrates over a period of time that eventually leaves the cells unresponsive to insulin (you've worn the receptors out). Eventually the pancreas rebels and no longer produces insulin. This is Type 2 diabetes and is a lifestyle condition brought on by poor diet, inactivity and being overweight.

An autoimmune disease of the pancreas gland where the body's immune system attacks and gradually destroys the gland. Eventually the gland can no longer produce insulin, and injections of insulin and regular blood glucose monitoring are required. This is Type 1 diabetes.

If you are experiencing any of the symptoms above, particularly excessive thirst and frequent urinating, you should consult your doctor immediately.

» Chronic stress and adrenal exhaustion

Is this you?

- You have trouble waking up and pulling yourself together to get up in the morning
- You have difficulty concentrating and focusing
- You need something like caffeine to get you going, and caffeine hits during the day to keep you on your feet

Part
1

- You often crave something salty, sweet or fatty
- You feel a bit better after lunch but then have a mid-afternoon energy crash
- You suddenly feel better about 6pm, and the feeling lasts until 9pm or 10pm... but then you're exhausted
- If you don't go to bed as soon as exhaustion hits, you may get a second wind which could keep you awake until 1 or 2 in the morning

If this is frequently your daily routine, there's a good chance you may be experiencing adrenal fatigue.

The adrenals are two tiny triangular-shaped glands attached to the top of each kidney. Their primary function is to enable you to deal with trauma, shock and danger. They are the central operator in the 'fight or flight' response and are critical for your survival. When danger is detected, and to be frank, this may well be caused by a sudden demand or a stressful situation, your adrenals are instructed by the brain to produce and release a whole cascade of hormones. These hormones will generate a variety of changes in the body to help you deal with the perceived danger. If you're going to fight or flee, energy is required – so the adrenals also play a role in energy management.

The problem, though, is that we have this mechanism to manage danger that comes and goes. In other words: you perceive danger, your adrenal hormones will prepare you to run or fight, the danger goes away, and the body returns to normal. Stimulating your body to generate the energy to save yourself is momentary, then calm resumes and you relax.

In today's crazy, highly demanding world, we're being bombarded with pressures, challenges, worries, shocks and upsets; and because your brain cannot distinguish what is life-threatening and what is not, it activates the stress response every time. This puts us in a state of chronic stress, which means our stress response becomes stuck in 'always-on' and we're constantly drawing on our energy reserves. We struggle to take the time to switch off and allow the body to relax, and because of this we're not giving our energy stores time to recharge. Our battery is running low.

If 'stress' is relentless and your capacity to remain in control and cope diminishes, your resilience is worn down, and the result is you could crash and burn out. Your energy is shot and you struggle to function. You've worn yourself out and it's utterly miserable. This topic is covered in more detail in Chapter 9 and in my best-selling book *How to Prevent Burnout*.

Activities to identify your energy zappers

Activity 1: Your energy audit

1. Choose a typical weekday to record your findings.
2. Record your energy levels each hour, on the hour. If you miss the hour, record the time you took a reading.
3. Score your energy, where 1 is the lowest you could have and 10 is very high.
4. Record what you were doing at the time. You could have been eating, exercising, answering emails, in a meeting, commuting. Whatever you were doing, write it down.
5. Repeat the exercise on two more days.

Energy is never consistent: even those of us flying high on energy will have some times in the day when we are really productive and other times when we are not fit to do anything at all. Feeling really energised can still change in intensity over the day, and people suffering underactive thyroid or adrenal fatigue symptoms will experience times in the day when their energy is appalling, and others when it is OK.

The aim of this exercise is to understand how your energy changes throughout your day. When you know this, it may help you to identify what is boosting and what is zapping your energy.

Time	Energy score	What you were doing

Look at your results to see whether there are any trends. You may always have more energy just after you have exercised or less when you are sitting at your desk. Record your answers below.

Part
1

Activity 2: What happens to you when your energy levels are running low?

Take yourself back to a time when you have felt very low on energy – or maybe that's now.

1. Think about every aspect of your life – physical, mental and emotional.
2. Think about your mood, emotions and behaviour. What signs did you, or do you, display?
3. Record your answers in the left-hand column.
4. In the right-hand column record how often these signs appear(ed): frequently, occasionally or rarely.

Signs that my energy is running low	Frequency

Activity 3: Nutrient robbers

1. Look at the diet and lifestyle factors below that can rob the nutrients in your body. Tick in the right-hand column which apply to you.
2. What changes could you make?

Nutrient robber	✓
Do you eat non-organic food?	
Do you store and eat your fruit and vegetables without washing?	
Do you use plastic water bottles more than once?	
Do you cook using plastic containers or cling film?	
Do you store food in plastic containers or cling film?	
Do you live in a city or by a road with heavy traffic?	
Do you regularly drive in heavy traffic?	
Do you smoke, or live with a heavy smoker who smokes in the house?	
Do you regularly use painkillers?	
Do you eat tuna fish?	
Do you drink alcohol more than three times a week?	
Have you had two or more prescriptions for antibiotics in the last twelve months?	

Activity 4: Nutrient deficiencies

In the next chart are the key nutrients required by the energy production cycle that can be deficient.

1. Look at the symptoms of deficiency identified for each nutrient.
2. Tick or underline the condition that is relevant to you now.
3. Record your findings in the reflections chart at the end of this chapter.

Magnesium	Iron
• Muscle tremors or cramp	• Anaemia
• Muscle pain	• Chronic fatigue or listlessness
• Restlessness	• Pale skin
• Anxiety	• Muscle weakness
• Difficulty sleeping	• Difficulty concentrating
• High blood pressure	• Difficulty remembering things
• Headaches or migraines	• Loss of appetite
• Irregular heartbeat	• Nausea
• Loss of appetite	• Sore tongue
• Constipation	• Heavy periods

Coenzyme Q10	Sulphur
• Extreme fatigue	• Low energy
• Muscle pain	• Muscle pain
• Muscle weakness	• Muscle weakness
• High cholesterol	• Dry, itchy scalp
• High blood pressure	• Acne
• Cardiovascular conditions	• Eczema or dermatitis
• Poor blood sugar balance	• Migraine headaches
• Gum disease	• Painful or irregular periods
• Headaches or migraines	• Stomach problems
• Frequent coughs or colds	• Sore throat

Vitamin B1: Thiamine	Vitamin B2: Riboflavin
• Muscle weakness	• Cracks in corner of mouth
• Tingling in hands and feet	• Chapped lips
• Prickly legs	• Mouth infections
• Tender muscles	• Throat swelling
• Involuntary eye movement	• Swollen tongue
• Loss of memory	• Unusual sensitivity to light
• Mental confusion	• Burning, gritty or watering eyes
• Irritability	• Bloodshot eyes
• Rapid heartbeat	• Easily fatigued
• Poor appetite	• Dermatitis

Vitamin B3: Niacin	Vitamin B5: Pantothenic acid
• Indigestion	• Exhaustion after light activity
• Diarrhoea	• Insomnia
• Vomiting	• Depression
• Fatigue	• Irritability
• Mouth ulcers	• Burning feet
• Depression	• Tender heals
• Irritability	• Stomach pains
• High cholesterol	• Nausea or vomiting
• Insomnia	• Muscle cramps
• Headaches or migraines	• Teeth grinding
Vitamin B6: Pyridoxine	**Vitamin B7: Biotin**
• Depression	• Fine or brittle hair
• Nervousness or anxiety	• Prematurely greying hair
• Confusion	• Hair loss
• Nausea	• Eczema or dermatitis
• Anaemia	• Dry skin
• Water retention	• Tender or sore muscles
• Frequent infections	• Loss of appetite
• Dermatitis	• Nausea
• Muscle pain	• Fatigue
• Premenstrual tension	• Depression
Vitamin B9: Folic acid	**Vitamin B12**
• Frequent infections	• Extreme fatigue
• Extreme fatigue	• Tingling in feet and hands
• Poor appetite	• Tender or sore muscles
• Constipation	• Irritability
• Anaemia	• Depression
• Mouth ulcers	• Sore or red tongue
• Swollen tongue	• Disturbed vision
• Irritability	• Depression
• Pale skin	• Problems with memory
• Prematurely greying hair	• Ringing in ears

Part
1

Now that you understand what burnout is, how it affects you and where you're at, let's move on to some ways of reflecting on your life and managing your situation. Remember, I did say that you *can* have your cake and eat it!

Read these carefully and choose the activities that are doable for you without causing you extra stress.

Activity 5: Your energisers and drainers

1. What and who *currently* are the things in your life that are good for you? Record everything you can think of in the Energisers column of the chart opposite. Consider diet, lifestyle, people, events, relationships, personal attitudes and beliefs.
Note: this is about what you have right now, not what you think you should have.

2. What and who are the things in your life that are bad for you, that drain you, stress you and spark off negative feelings and emotions? Record these in the Drainers column.

3. If there is something you think could be recorded in both columns, put it in both, but try to identify the difference that makes it either an energiser or a drainer overall.

4. Mark the top five items in each column and rank them from one to five.

5. Look at the Drainers column and reflect on the following questions:

• Why are these drainers so significant?

• What specific aspect of each drainer is draining you?

• What impact are these drainers having on your life?

• What can you do to diminish the impact of drainers or remove them completely from your life?

The reality is that you have three choices to improve your life.

- To take action and change the situation.
- To change yourself to adapt, for example by reframing how you perceive things.
- To accept the situation and ignore it.

6. What can you do to have more of the energisers in your life?

Energisers	Drainers

Your reflections

What has resonated with you while reading about energy zappers?
- What have you learned about yourself?
- What have you learned about what may be zapping you of energy?
- What do you need to start doing that you have not done before?
- What other thoughts do you have?

PART 2

The 7 steps to optimum energy

CHAPTER 3

The 7 Steps to Optimum Energy model

How much do you know about energy?

◊ Do you find it difficult to articulate what 'personal energy' actually means?

◊ Are you tired of feeling tired all the time and don't know what to do about it?

◊ Is low energy becoming a barrier to your performance?

◊ Do you know how your body and mind make energy?

When you have energy, you feel fantastic! You are happier, more productive and creative.

In physics, energy is described as the capacity to do work. In humans it's much, much more than that. *Energy is your vitality and your capacity to live life*. It's with you 24/7. You wake up with it and you go to bed with it, and it sees you through the night while you sleep. It's the very fuel in your tank that drives your motivation and capability to bring your skills and talents to life and achieve what you want to achieve. It's the essence of living.

So, no matter how much we plan and prioritise tasks, we can

only perform them effectively if we have the energy to do them. Energy is the fundamental currency of high performance and if we use it without replenishment, we will be physically, mentally and emotionally fatigued. This affects our concentration, mood, memory, creativity and performance.

Renewing and recharging energy is, therefore, imperative because humans can only perform at their best when they rhythmically cycle between energy expenditure and energy renewal. Energy comes primarily from the food we eat and a finely balanced hormone system, but this isn't the whole story. Our mind, emotions, spirit and sense of purpose have an enormous influence on it too.

The **7 Steps to Optimum Energy** model embraces all of these elements: Nutrition, Sleep, Movement, Connectivity, Purpose, Balance and Positivity.

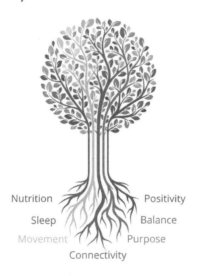

Nutrition

Sleep

Movement

Connectivity

Positivity

Balance

Purpose

Part 2

Each chapter in this book is devoted to a particular step to optimum energy. Don't be tempted to cherry-pick your favourite. There is a quote by Alfred Lord Tennyson: "I am a part of all that I have met." Your energy is the sum of many parts; of everything your mind and body come into contact with. Revitalising your mind with social connections, a sense of purpose, positive thinking and managing stress is just as important as energising your body with food, sleep and movement. The real power comes when they are all optimised. They work in harmony, invigorating your very physical, mental, emotional and spiritual being and strengthening your resilience. Energy is a mind and body thing!

Let me just remind you of the description I provided for each of these steps in the Introduction.

Step 1: Nutrition. This is the most basic requirement. Virtually every cell in your body contains little energy factories called mitochondria which primarily use blood glucose and a variety of nutrients to generate energy. Unless you are well nourished, nothing else will be able to optimise your energy.

Step 2: Sleep. You cannot function without sleep. You have evolved to use this time to restore, repair and recover from the strains of your time awake. You need good-quality sleep in sufficient quantity. If sleep is compromised, so is your energy.

Step 3: Movement. This is a vital component of the energy production process. Exercise increases oxygen to your cells and clears carbon dioxide from them.

Step 4: Connectivity. People need people. We're social animals and we get so much of our energy from connecting with other people. Connecting with others makes you happy and engaged and can help you to switch off from the internal chatter that's exacerbating the stress you feel.

Step 5: Purpose. Purpose is your inner self, your spirit, the very energy that drives you. Knowing what's important to you, following your direction in life and living that dream feed your sense of meaning and generate energy.

Step 6: Balance. Life can be stressful. Your body's mechanism for managing these challenges is to go into 'fight or flight' mode and release two hormones: adrenalin and cortisol. If you are leading a fast-paced, highly demanding life, you could be stuck in an 'always-on', high-stress-hormone state, and this will put huge demands on your energy.

Step 7: Positivity. Positivity is about the positive emotions that energise and motivate you. As part of your survival mechanism, you will be on alert for danger and this creates negative thinking pathways in your brain, which in turn lowers mood. Positivity creates chemicals in your brain that improve your outlook and energise you.

The next two exercises will help you to identify which sections are the most important for optimising your personal energy. Your days and evenings are full, so it might feel daunting to think that you need to do everything suggested in this book. If you do too much, it will just exhaust you and demotivate you, and your life of low energy will continue as the norm. By prioritising the actions you need to incorporate into your lifestyle, you will give yourself the best chance of being successful.

Part 2

Activity 1: The Energy Risk Factors Questionnaire
1. Read the statements in the next chart and put a tick in the column that honestly reflects you and your lifestyle right now.
2. Add up your score for each column.

	Is this you?	Never	Rarely	Some-times	Often	Always
1	Is your eating sporadic and unplanned, grabbing food when you can?					
2	Do you skip at least one meal a day more than twice a week?					
3	Do you crave sweet, sugary things – cake, biscuits, chocolate, toast and honey?					
4	Do you rely on tea or coffee or caffeine drinks or cigarettes to give you a lift?					
5	Do you use food just as fuel, and not give the time to thinking about nutrition?					
6	Do you find your moods are bad when you haven't eaten for a while?					
7	Do you eat 'on the go'?					
8	Do you have difficulty getting to sleep or staying asleep?					
9	Do you stay up late (after 11pm)?					
10	Do you set your alarm for earlier so you can get up and get more done?					
11	Are you on your smartphone, laptop or tablet up to one hour before you climb into bed?					
12	Do you do some competitive sport up to two hours before you go to bed?					
13	Do you avoid exercise because you feel too tired?					
14	Do you slump on the sofa watching mindless TV in the evening?					

Part
2

	Is this you?	Never	Rarely	Some-times	Often	Always
15	Is your diary too crazy to allow any time for exercise?					
16	Do you find it hard to find the time to switch off and relax?					
17	Do you feel guilty when relaxing?					
18	Do you have to force yourself to keep going rather than take a quick break?					
19	Do you have a persistent need for achievement?					
20	Are you especially competitive?					
21	Do you like things to be perfect with no mistakes?					
22	Do you work independently, preferring not to ask someone for help?					
23	Do you feel as if your 'to-do' list never gets any shorter?					
24	Do you find it difficult to say 'no' and end up over-committing yourself?					
25	Do you feel as if your time is over-committed?					
26	Do you feel you're doing more and more but you're the only one who can do it?					
27	Do you avoid people in case they ask you to do something for them?					
28	Do you talk over people or finish their sentence to speed things up?					
29	Are you frequently checking for emails and phone messages?					
30	Are you often doing two or three tasks simultaneously?					

Part 2

	Is this you?	Never	Rarely	Some-times	Often	Always
31	Does it seem too much effort to see friends and socialise?					
32	Do you find your memory gets foggy periodically during the day?					
33	Do you find you don't have much enthusiasm for anything?					
34	Do you feel people are a nuisance and irritate you?					
35	Do you find it hard to concentrate and think creatively?					
36	Are you unclear about your purpose in life?					
37	Do you find it hard to relate to people?					
38	Do you feel as though your life is defined by your work right now?					
39	Do you rarely experience great joy, love or happiness?					
40	Do you find yourself staring into the air?					
41	Have you stopped confiding in friends and family?					
42	Do you rarely pay compliments to others?					
Total score						

The items in this questionnaire are the activities that put you at risk of draining your energy. The more ticks you have in the 'Often' and 'Always' columns, the more your energy may be compromised and the higher risk that you may become extremely fatigued or even burn out.

Look carefully at these items, as they will give you clues as to what activities you can undertake to improve your energy.

3. Record in the box below the statements that are of most concern to you. These could be light-bulb moments which have highlighted what may be the underlying cause of your low energy, or statements that you know about but have not done anything to correct.

When you're feeling low on energy, struggling to cope, feeling stressed or overwhelmed, it can help you to take yourself back to this time and draw on these feelings.

Invite a memory back from a time when you felt full of energy and vitality. Answer the following questions.

Use this exercise to identify the aspects of your life that generate energy. Is it feeling well fed, having slept well, feeling calm or maybe doing what's important to you? This may help you to focus the sections and activities required to optimise your personal energy.

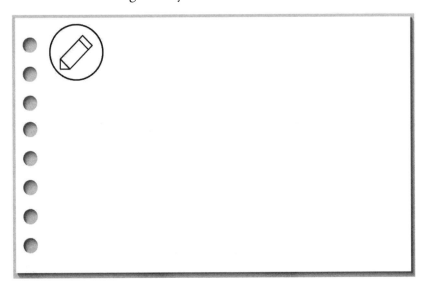

Activity 2: When you were energised

1. Imagine you are looking at yourself from the outside. What do you look like physically and how are you acting?
2. How does it feel to be so energised? What feelings and emotions arise?
3. What is it that's actually making you feel so full of energy and act with such vitality? Try to dig as deep as you can to identify the source of your energy.

Your reflections

What has resonated with you while reading this introduction to the '7 Steps to Optimum Energy Model'?

- What have you learned about yourself?
- What have you learned about the state of your energy?
- What have you learned about the reasons for your low energy?
- What do you need to start doing that you have not done before?
- What other thoughts do you have?

Part 2

CHAPTER 4

Step 1: Nutrition for optimum energy

◊ Do you find it hard to concentrate at times during the day?

◊ Do you grab food on the run to give you a quick energy boost?

◊ Do you need tea and/or coffee and/or cola to keep you going throughout the day?

◊ Do you find you're drinking more alcohol during the evenings and at weekends?

◊ Do you experience sugar cravings?

◊ Do you experience mood swings?

◊ Does the thought of eating breakfast fill you with horror?

I f you have answered "Yes" to any of these questions, you need to pay extra special attention to this section.

The saying "You are what you eat" is so true. Just as your car would splutter and grind to a halt if you filled it up with the wrong fuel, so your body will do the same. It's all about the quality of the fuel you use.

Today's low-nutrient, heavily processed, carbohydrate- and stimulant-loaded diet does provide the calories we need to function, but only at a basic level. If you want to fly through life with focus and vitality, you need fuelling up in a way that allows you to thrive. That means fuel that both ensures your engine runs smoothly and cleans it along the way. You know the petrol adverts tell you that their brand has all the qualities your car needs? Well it's the same for your mind and body. But rather than consuming a petrochemical, you should be fuelling yourself up, and keeping yourself topped up throughout the day, on a rich and varied diet of fresh, nutrient-dense foods.

Scoffing and snacking on processed, highly refined food will eventually wreck your engine. One minute you'll be firing on all cylinders, and the next crashing and craving a quick fix of something sweet and carbohydrate-rich to lift you back up again.

If you want to live a life full of energy and vitality, the best place to start is with what you eat. Food **is** the fuel of life. Without it, you wouldn't stand any chance of functioning. Fail to address your nutritional needs and nothing else in this book will give you the effect you're looking for.

Part 2

That's because eating well improves the health of your digestive tract and the quality of your digestion so you are able to break down and absorb the nutrients you need. It balances your blood sugar levels and energy levels and nourishes those tiny powerhouses in your cells, your mitochondria, without which you wouldn't be able to produce energy.

That's why, despite a successful career as a psychologist, I spent three years studying to become a nutritionist. Attitudes, emotions, feelings and behaviour are heavily influenced by the health of your brain. I believe that brain health starts with fuelling it in the right way. Get it right and it functions well. Get it wrong and the toxicity has a detrimental effect.

John's story

John was a senior business executive who suffered constantly from acid reflux. He felt dreadful. He had powerful stomach pains and burning sensations in his chest, and struggled with energy. His job meant that he would be eating at irregular times, often taking in protein (especially meat) late at night and then going to sleep full and bloated.

To counteract the symptoms, he was guzzling antacid medication, bought from his local pharmacy in large quantities and frequently. While this would give some short-term relief, he found that the symptoms would soon start again and the cycle continue.

The short-term answer is paradoxical – the real reason for John's problem was not too much stomach acid, but too little! John was struggling to digest his food, particularly the heavy red meat he favoured late in the evening. It was very likely that this lack of stomach acid prevented the release and absorption of the very nutrients required to make stomach acid: a circle of destruction.

What John needed to do was to increase the amount of stomach acid when he ate, so that his stomach would digest the food more rapidly.

I set him up with some digestive enzyme supplements specifically designed to support the stomach: HCI and Pepsin. He took these with each meal and almost immediately symptoms reduced, and then he could begin to make more fundamental changes to his diet and eating patterns.

This included being more careful about what he was eating – reducing the amount of heavy red meat and hard cheese, and adding more fish to his diet, which is easier to digest. He increased his vegetable and fruit intake and added more complex carbohydrates to his diet to increase fibre and the nutrients required to produce stomach acid, in particular zinc.

He also changed his eating patterns, to ensure he had three decent meals a day, and small snacks between breakfast and lunch and between

Part
2

lunch and dinner. He ensured that dinner was eaten before 8pm, and that he then fasted until about 8am the next morning.

Of course, with his hectic schedule, this didn't always work; but even when he broke with his plan, he was sufficiently aware of the consequences to ensure he took care with his diet.

As a result, he no longer, or only very rarely, has to resort to digestive enzyme supplements. His energy levels are greater, and the absence of pain has also given him the 'space' to take up other energy-enhancing activities with further benefits to his life.

If you need to make alterations to your diet that will improve the health of your digestive tract and fuel up your mitochondria, read on. There are seven steps for you to follow that help you fuel up in the best possible way.

Part 2

1.   Feed your mitochondria

We've already been introduced to our extraordinary little engines in our cells, our mitochondria; and we know that to create units of energy, mitochondria rely primarily on *glucose* plus a variety of vitamins and minerals, as well as oxygen, to drive the chemical conversion of glucose into energy.

Glucose comes from *carbohydrate* foods. These are starchy foods, such as bread, pasta, rice, potatoes, lentils and bananas, along with sugar found in table sugar, maple syrup, honey and fruit.

When we eat carbohydrates, whether they be starch or sugar, our digestive system breaks them down into simple molecules of glucose, which are then absorbed into the bloodstream and transported to the cells around our body ready for the mitochondria to work their magic.

Not all carbohydrates are the same, though. Modern food

processing has meant that we now have two types to fuel up on – those in their natural form, which we call *complex carbohydrates*; and the carbohydrates that the food industry has stripped of their fibre, which we call *simple carbohydrates*. Complex carbohydrates include wholewheat flour, oats and brown rice. Simple carbohydrates include white bread, white pasta, white rice and sugar.

Let's look a bit further into the energy production process. Each cell absorbs the glucose, then converts it into a molecule for the mitochondria to put through a series of chemical processes, which eventually produce energy. This conversion engine requires a variety of vitamin and mineral nutrients to fuel it. We cannot make these nutrients ourselves – we only get them from food. They are released from our food as we digest it and then absorbed into the bloodstream to be taken to our cells. For the conversion to work efficiently, a variety of vitamins and minerals are needed, and this is why a nutritious diet is fundamental if you're going to optimise your energy. It's no good having the ingredients if you haven't got the components of the machine to manufacture energy.

Consuming just simple carbohydrates will not provide you with high-grade, sustainable energy. The cells cannot utilise them efficiently, and instead store them as fat for use another time if necessary.

Mitochondria are amazing! Something so tiny gives us all we need to live our lives. It's not a simple process, though. Glucose is taken through a three-step, nutrient-demanding process. If you're interested in the science, here is how the process works:

Step One is *glycolysis*. This takes place in the cell's cytoplasm, and is where glucose is converted into pyruvate and a very small amount of adenosine triphosphate (ATP), the energy molecule. Two minerals, magnesium and phosphorus, are required for this process to work properly.

Part
2

Step Two takes place in the matrix of the mitochondria and is called the *citric acid cycle*. It converts the pyruvate produced by glycolysis into acetyl CoA. With a complex series of chemical reactions using oxygen, acetyl CoA is converted into carbon dioxide, electrically charged molecules called *NADH* and *FADH2*, and a small amount of energy (ATP).

This complex process needs an array of nutrients, including the B vitamins (B1, B2, B3, B5) and the minerals manganese, magnesium, iron, sulphur and phosphorus.

Step Three sees the electrically charged NADH and FADH2 release their hydrogen electrons into the electron transport chain in the inner membrane of the mitochondria. This is the most complex part of the process – but also the most productive, as the flow of electrons across the membrane produces the most ATP by far during this three-step process (thirty-four of the thirty-eight molecules of ATP energy). The process requires the minerals iron, copper and phosphorus, plus Coenzyme Q10, which is similar to a vitamin.

When glucose from carbohydrates is in short supply, which would happen if you exercised for more than an hour or you preferred a low-carbohydrate diet, proteins and fats can be broken down and used by the Krebs cycle.

I've highlighted how nutrient-demanding this three-step process is. Nature is very clever: these nutrients are primarily found in fibre-rich complex carbohydrates – wholegrains, green leafy vegetables, beans and fruit. You get all you need in one package! I would always advise you boost this further with at least one very colourful meal that will provide you with a burst of nutrients. Eat these, instead of simple carbohydrates, and your energy will be much more sustainable to manage even during the times you are resting or sleeping, because you still need to keep your heart pumping, maintain your breathing, and allow your liver to detox and your kidneys to filter. Without this energy, you'll feel hungry and will be waking in the night with the munchies, disturbing your sleep cycle.

I mentioned earlier that food production processes are stripping out the nutrients in our food. Food farming is doing the same. The high demand for food means the soil no longer contains the levels of nutrients it used to. This means grains and vegetables do not contain anywhere near the level of nutrients they did fifty years ago. A varied, colourful diet ensures that you obtain all the nutrients you need from a variety of sources. However, there are some nutrients I find the population is often low in, and these are B vitamins, magnesium and iron. Taking statins for high cholesterol can inhibit the absorption of Coenzyme Q10, which is why so many people on statins have muscular aches.

Take a look at the table below to see what foods you could include in your diet to ensure you're getting all you need to meet your energy demand.

Part 2

Nutrient and activity	Food source
Complex carbohydrate: Broken down by digestion into glucose, the fuel for mitochondria Also contains vitamins and minerals essential for producing energy	• Wholegrains – wheat, rye, barley, oats • Green vegetables – broccoli, kale, courgette, green beans, watercress, rocket, spinach • Orange vegetables – sweet potato, carrots • Fruit, particularly berries
Protein: Can be broken down by the body into ammonia to provide fuel for energy High in nutrients	• Lean meat – chicken, turkey, game, lamb, beef • Fish, seafood • Dairy products – milk, cheese, yoghurt, cottage cheese • Beans, lentils, quinoa

Fat: Can be broken down by the body into ketones to provide a fuel for energy production if glucose is in short supply Good oils assist the transport of glucose across the cell wall	• Oily fish – salmon, trout, mackerel, fresh tuna (not tinned) • Nuts – Brazil nuts, almonds, walnuts • Seeds – sunflower, pumpkin, sesame, hemp, chia, flax • Omega-3 eggs • Coconut
Vitamin B complex: Important throughout the energy production cycle	• Green leafy vegetables (broccoli, kale, Brussels sprouts, spinach), wheatgerm, wholegrains, mushrooms, eggs, nuts and seeds
Key minerals – magnesium, manganese, iron: Required for the energy formation cycle	• Magnesium: green leafy vegetables, almonds, pumpkin seeds • Manganese: greens, squash, corn, tomatoes, onions, aubergine, mushrooms • Phosphorus: wholegrain cereals, milk, fish, grapes • Iron: fortified cereals, beef, shellfish, dried apricots, beans and lentils, dark green leafy vegetables, pumpkin seeds
Coenzyme Q10: Required to spark oxygen in the energy furnace and protecting the cell from energy production by-products	• Lean meat, oily fish, walnuts, peanuts, pistachios, sesame seeds, broccoli, cauliflower, orange, strawberries

Be aware of what you eat and how food makes you feel. Food intolerances and allergies may create inflammation in the gut and have the potential to reduce the way you absorb your food. You might be eating well, but your body may not be gaining any of the benefits. If you suspect a food intolerance, cut one suspect food out of your diet for two weeks and see how you feel when you reintroduce it. Never cut more than one food type out at a time. The most common intolerances are wheat (gluten), dairy (lectins), yeast and soya. Food intolerances frequently affect energy.

2.   Balance your blood sugar

The blood sugar rollercoaster

We've explored the reasons why an unprocessed diet is the way to go, but the frequency of your meals matters just as much as the food you consume. If your meals are irregular or not as healthy as you may think they are, you will put yourself on the blood sugar rollercoaster. It goes like this.

Your body needs a sustainable source of energy on which it can draw as and when it needs to. As we have seen, energy comes from glucose, which is transported to the body's cells and used on demand. The speed with which the bloodstream absorbs from the digestive system has a big impact on our energy's sustainability. Gaining energy is not about eating as much carbohydrate as you can – it's about eating the correct carbohydrate at the correct pace. It's about eating the right type of carbohydrates which can be broken down in the digestive system and absorbed into the bloodstream in a slow and steady manner rather than a frantic rush.

When glucose is absorbed into the bloodstream, it stimulates insulin, a hormone that helps to transport glucose into the cells. As too much glucose can be toxic for the cells and brain, your body has a finely tuned feedback mechanism that warns it if the glucose level rises too high.

When there's too much glucose in the bloodstream, the feedback mechanism stimulates the releases of extra insulin. This takes the extra glucose to the liver for storage, and any further excess to be converted to fat and stored. The very act of doing this reduces the amount of glucose in the bloodstream significantly; in fact, it takes it down so fast that you feel low on energy again.

When levels are low, you crave foods that will give you a quick surge of energy again – typically refined carbohydrates which are quickly broken down and absorbed into the bloodstream. This shoots blood glucose levels up to a level higher than required, and so insulin again

Part
2

appears to correct things… and then your energy drops, so you crave anything that will give you a quick boost again.

It's like if you hit the accelerator hard but your body then hits the brakes hard, so you respond by hitting the accelerator hard again and your body hits the brakes hard again, and so it goes on… and you become more and more tired, which stresses your body more and more… so, on top of this, your adrenals are being over-stimulated.

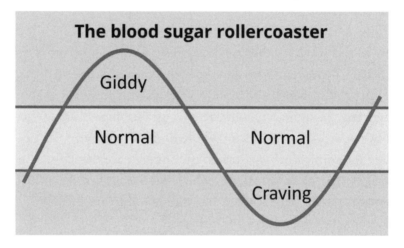

The blood sugar rollercoaster

Giddy

Normal

Normal

Craving

These highs and lows in blood sugar mean that nothing quite knows whether it is coming or going – including you – and that's because you've taken a ride on the *blood sugar rollercoaster*, which, despite its name, is no fun at all.

Look at the chart opposite for the signs of high and low blood sugar. When blood glucose is high…

- You feel giddy and heady.
- It may be difficult to focus.
- The frequent stimulation of insulin puts you at risk of Type 2 diabetes.
- Your clothes don't fit as you're storing more fat (particularly around the middle).
- You experience mood swings.

When blood sugar is low…

- You crave stimulants and quick-fix, high-glucose foods.
- You feel tired and grumpy.
- Your body produces stress hormones which create further imbalances in your blood sugar.

High blood sugar	Balanced blood sugar	Low blood sugar
• Buzzing • Hyper • Fast thinking • Agitated • Hard to focus • Feel 'heady'	• Energised • Able to focus • Good concentration • Good mood • Good recollection and memory • Original, creative thinking	• Feel faint and weak • Mood swings – grumpy, snappy • Difficulty concentrating • Poor memory • Energy slump during the day • Needing stimulants to keep going • Craving something sweet

Part 2

Not all carbohydrates are the same

We've seen how complex carbohydrates contain the nutrients you require for energy production – but there's another advantage, which is the fibre they contain. Fibre slows the digestion of carbohydrates, which means the absorption of glucose takes place at a slower, steady pace, sustaining your energy for longer – unlike with simple carbohydrates, which are like rocket fuel. Other carbohydrate foods, such as beans and lentils, also contain protein which takes longer to digest and so slows absorption.

Fruit contains a slower-release form of glucose called *fructose*, which is easily absorbed but has to make a visit to the liver on the way to your cells to convert it to glucose.

The message here is that to get off this ghastly rollercoaster ride, you need to create a more sustainable balance in blood sugar levels. This starts with diet:

- Eating the right type of carbohydrates, which can be broken down in the digestive system and absorbed into the bloodstream in a slow and steady manner rather than a frantic rush.
- Including in your meal other foods, such as protein and fat, that slow the breakdown of carbohydrate food further and keep your energy levels steady for longer. This would include lean meat, oily fish, eggs, cheese, yoghurt, chickpeas, lentils, whey protein powder, nuts and seeds.
- Between meals, have a nutrient-dense snack if your energy is flagging – not a processed and sugary biscuit or cake. A small serving of nuts, including Brazil, walnut, or almonds, or pumpkin seeds, will provide a vast array of nutrients required for the energy production process.

Here are a few tips on how to prevent taking the 'blood sugar rollercoaster' ride

Always eat breakfast. Your body has been fasting for ten to twelve hours and needs glucose, otherwise it stimulates the stress response. If you can't face anything first thing, have something when you get to work and always eat before 10am.

Plan your meals in advance and use leftovers from the previous evening's meal for lunch, rather than buying a sandwich.

Make time to eat and don't get hungry! You need to eat regularly to balance your blood sugar. Eat three meals a day and have a small snack in the morning and afternoon.

Avoid adding sugar to your food or drink – sugar provides empty calories. If you add sugar to your tea or coffee, gradually reduce it each week until you have none.

Reduce the amount of fruit juice and fruit smoothies you drink (apple, orange, pineapple, even freshly squeezed orange juice). Smoothies are worse than natural fruit because they have had the fibre removed, so the sugar is quickly absorbed. Initially, dilute any fruit drinks until you can eventually give them up.

Avoid foods with added sugar. 'Healthy' snack bars, free-from foods, low-fat foods, tinned soups, baked beans, sauces and fruit yoghurt are often laden with sugar to provide flavour.

Avoid all energy drinks, including cola, which contain caffeine and sugar. A double whammy. Energy drinks often contain caffeine to give a boost but seriously affect blood sugar balance.

Check labels. When you buy ready-made food products, check the label for sugar content. Avoid foods with anything over 5g of sugar per 100g of food. Five grams is equivalent to one teaspoon.

Part 2

Avoid artificial sweeteners found in low-calorie drinks. Artificial sweeteners trick the body into thinking we've had something sweet when we haven't. We therefore crave sugar and look elsewhere to get it. As a result, we can end up eating far more of it. Such products confuse the body and stress it.

Avoid alcohol or keep your intake to the minimum. It's high in sugar!

Here are some of the important nutrients your body needs to help you balance blood sugar, together with suggestions about which foods contain them.

Helpful foods to prevent the blood sugar rollercoaster

Nutrient	Where to find it
Chromium	• Turkey, eggs • Whole foods, brown rice, flour, bread and pasta • Beans, nuts, seeds, almonds, chia • Asparagus, mushrooms, apple, banana, green beans
Magnesium	Wheatgerm, almonds, chia, pumpkin seeds, green vegetables
B vitamins	Wheatgerm, fish, fruit and vegetables, wholegrains, mushrooms, eggs

Helpful supplements if you want to get off the blood sugar rollercoaster

You can also consider the following supplements:

Part 2

Nutrient	What it does	What to take
Chromium	Helpful for insulin and blood sugar management. Helps you to manage sugar cravings. It is a vital ingredient of *glucose tolerance factor*, the hormone-like compound that works with insulin to transport glucose from blood into the cells.	400–600mcg per day of chromium picolinate or polynicotinate (better absorbed). Take in morning to balance blood sugar.
Magnesium	Plays a role in carbohydrate metabolism, so helps to regulate blood sugar levels.	500mg once a day with food.
B vitamins	Important for carbohydrate metabolism. B3 (non-flush niacin) helps control blood sugar levels.	Take a B complex plus 30mg niacinamide B3 (make sure it is non-skin flushing).

3.   Reduce your stimulant intake

We meet our craving for energy by consuming stimulants such as tea and coffee, alcohol, cigarettes and recreational drugs.

Coffee, tea, cigarettes and drugs contain no calories, so there is no way they'll provide you with any energy. It's all an illusion! What they do is to make you *think* they're energising you. They do this in two ways.

- They stimulate your liver to release stored glucose. This requires the release of stress hormones (adrenalin and cortisol), which means you put yourself into a state of stress – this isn't good for your health, and uses up more energy in the long run.
- They stimulate the release of *dopamine* in the brain – a chemical that improves your mood and gives you a sense of reward. It feels wonderful for a short time, but soon wears off, leaving you craving for more.

The best thing you can do is to identify the stimulants you rely on to boost your energy and avoid or considerably reduce them.

If it's coffee or strong tea, you'll need to wean yourself off it gradually. They contain caffeine, so do this by reducing your daily intake – otherwise you may find you get a headache or feel groggy. If you have five cups of coffee a day, cut out one cup and drink only the four cups for one week, then cut another cup out.

Be careful what you replace your drink with. If at all possible, make it a glass of filtered water, but should you prefer a hot drink, look for tea and coffee alternatives such as fruit and herb teas or natural coffee alternatives. Rooibos tea (redbush tea) is popular because you can add milk to it. Moringa tea also contains nutrients to boost energy, but make sure you use a caffeine-free brand. Decaffeinated tea will not do the job. The caffeine may have been stripped out, but it still contains two stimulating chemicals.

Part
2

Green tea is high in caffeine, so avoid it until you have built up your energy levels, and use it as part of your maintenance programme.

Cut back on alcohol, and avoid it completely at lunchtime. Although it might initially make you feel happy and relaxed, alcohol actually contains high amounts of sugar, which disrupts your blood sugar balance, leaving you craving a high-energy fix.

Quit smoking. The chemicals in cigarettes drain your nutrient reserves, and your nutrients are precious commodities if you want to produce real energy.

Give some thought to *why* you rely on certain nutrients. What changes can you make to reduce the stimulus? See the exercises at the end of this chapter for some guidance.

4.   Stay well hydrated

Around 60 per cent of the adult body is water, so it's vital to maintain hydration. Dehydration affects our cells' capability to generate energy, particularly in the brain. It's frequently the case that when I see people struggling to function, it's actually because they haven't had enough to drink. If you wait until you're thirsty to drink, it means you're already dehydrated.

The best thing you can do to prevent dehydration is to drink small amounts of fluid regularly. You'll know whether you're drinking enough by the colour of your urine. It should be pale yellow in colour. If it's dark yellow, you're dehydrated.

Thinking you're hungry, when in fact you have been eating, can also be down to thirst. You'd be much better off having a drink than more food.

You should be drinking one and a half litres of water gradually over the course of a day (or roughly eight glasses). If you haven't been one to drink much, build this up gradually, otherwise you'll upset your body's electrolyte balance, which could leave you feeling dizzy and bloated.

To avoid being dehydrated, start the day by drinking some water when you first wake in the morning. You would have lost a significant amount of fluid during the night, particularly when the nights are warmer.

Keep a large glass or bottle of filtered water topped up on your desk during the day and sip it regularly. Avoid refilling used plastic water bottles. If you dislike the taste of water (the chlorine in tap water is ghastly, which is why it is best to drink filtered water), you can add a squeeze of lemon or lime to give it some flavour. Take the bottle of water with you to meetings.

5. Nurture your thyroid gland

As mentioned in Chapter 2, the thyroid gland is a butterfly-shaped gland in your neck which plays an important role in regulating your metabolism, heat generation, macro nutrient synthesis (protein, carbohydrate and fats), muscle control and heart function.

The gland primarily produces thyroxine, more commonly referred to as T4 – an inactive hormone which is released into the bloodstream, then converted to the active form, triiodothyronine or T3, by the liver and kidneys. The gland does also produce small amounts of the active T3, but it primarily relies on conversion.

You cannot achieve optimum energy without a properly performing thyroid gland. It plays a vital role in cellular respiration, the process of converting glucose and oxygen into ATP (energy) by regulating how glucose is converted into pyruvate, the first stage of the three-stage glycolysis process.

If your thyroid gland is under-functioning, it will not be producing enough thyroxine to support glycolysis (Stage One); and if Stage One falters, then so do the next two stages. This leaves you exhausted. Under-energised cells do not function properly, which means you'll experience a variety of symptoms across your mind and body, including everything from hair loss and dry skin to brain fog and the inability to conceive. It's a very powerful hormone, and if it is under-functioning you will feel it in so many different ways.

Not only do thyroid hormones affect cellular respiration: they also influence peristalsis in the gut (the movement of food through the gut) and digestive juice secretion. This means an under-performing thyroid gland limits your ability to break down and absorb nutrients, including the ones you need for energy production. It's a double whammy and why I had to cover this topic in this book. I suffer (and I really do suffer) from an underactive thyroid gland due to an autoimmune condition. It is a vast topic which can only be explored briefly for now.

The health of the gland is affected by poor diet, by immune dysfunction (as in my case), where your body attacks the gland and gradually kills the cells, and by chronic stress. Chronic stress

is particularly important to note because the thyroid gland requires the amino acid tyrosine and an assortment of nutrients, such as B vitamins, vitamin C, selenium and zinc, to produce thyroxine. It's the same for the adrenal glands. They also require tyrosine and these nutrients to produce stress hormones triggered by the 'fight or flight' response. As this 'fight or flight' response plays the main role in our ability to survive, your body will prioritise stress hormone production over thyroid hormone production and the conversion of T4 to T3.

This means that if you're very stressed, you need to work as hard as you can to up your nutrient intake. This is tough when you feel awful from managing all the pressures and demands on you.

Nutrition is important for three aspects of thyroid health:

- the synthesis of thyroid hormones
- the conversion of T4 to T3
- the sensitivity of receptor sites on the cell wall, to receive the thyroid hormone and transfer it through the cell membrane.

The synthesis of thyroid hormones

The synthesis of thyroid hormones by the thyroid gland is heavily dependent on tyrosine and iodine. Tyrosine comes from the conversion of the amino acid L-phenylalanine in the body. Amino acids are found in proteins, as identified in the box below. Iodine is a mineral, often associated with the sea. Tyrosine and iodine can be taken as supplements, but I would never recommend this without specialist clinical advice, because having too much can have the opposite effect and inhibit the thyroid gland.

A variety of other nutrients including selenium, iron, manganese, zinc, B vitamins and vitamin C act as co-factors, assisting the manufacture of the hormone. This is yet another reason for ensuring you have a healthy, varied diet.

Nutrient	Food source
Tyrosine	A diet rich in good-quality proteins – meat, fish, eggs, dairy, avocados, pumpkin seeds, cashew nuts, almonds, bananas, quinoa, beans and pulses
Iodine	Milk, fish, kelp, iodised salt, onions, radishes, mushrooms, egg white and cheese

Part 2

The conversion of T4 to T3

The conversion of T4 to T3 requires the enzyme 5'-deiodinase, which contains the mineral selenium. Brazil nuts are the best source of selenium, but beware: too much selenium can have the opposite effect by interfering with zinc bioavailability and reducing tissue iron stores. Low T3 and low iron are both implicated in low energy. Limit Brazil nuts to no more than four a day.

The levels of selenium, magnesium and zinc in our food have dropped over the years due to farming methods, and much of the population is deficient. Another nutrient required is copper, and deficiency is rare – particularly if you use contraceptive pills or HRT, as these elevate copper at the expense of zinc.

Goitrogens are naturally occurring substances found in certain foods – broccoli, sprouts, cauliflower, cabbage, kale, spinach, soybeans, peanuts, millet and strawberries. They are thought to block iodine utilisation, but research on this topic is mixed and changing. More recently, the advice has changed to avoiding these foods in their raw form. However, these foods are so nutritious (great sources of vitamin B and magnesium) that I still encourage including them in the diet: just don't eat too much raw.

Certain industrial and household toxins, such as polychlorinated biphenyl (PCBs), lead, mercury, chlorine in swimming pools, and fluoride in water and toothpaste, are considered to inhibit the conversion of T4 to T3. It is thought that they compete with the absorption of iodine.

And we shouldn't ignore the effect food intolerances and allergies can have on the gut and the absorption of key nutrients.

High levels of stress and extreme dieting also hinder the conversion of T4 to T3. If chronic stress is a fact of life for you, you may require additional adrenal support. I have found the herb rhodiola helpful, as it lowers elevated cortisol levels and improves the conversion of T4 to T3. There is much more about this in my book *How to Prevent Burnout*.

Nutrient	Food source
Selenium	Brazil nuts, garlic, onions, corn, kale, cabbage, broccoli, egg yolks, wheatgerm
Magnesium	Green leafy vegetables, fruit and nuts
Zinc	Oysters, red meat, egg yolks and fish
Copper	Prawns, oysters, nuts, avocados, mushrooms and green leafy vegetables

Sensitivity of the cell wall

The sensitivity of the receptor sites on the cell wall is improved by zinc and regular exercise. Omega 3 fats assist in the transport of T3 through the cell wall into the cytoplasm, ready to support glycolysis. Goitrogens are thought to inhibit receptor activity as well, as discussed above.

Nutrient	Food source
Zinc	Good-quality proteins – meat, fish, eggs, dairy, quinoa, beans and pulses
Omega 3 oils	Oily fish, nuts and seeds
Manganese	Green leafy vegetables, squash, pumpkin seeds, flax seeds, garlic, onions, mushrooms

Testing for thyroid function

It can be difficult to determine whether your low energy or exhaustion is due to an under-performing thyroid gland or an over-performing adrenal gland. Although both impact each other, and there is a chance it's both, here are a few clues to which it is.

Signs/symptoms	Adrenal	Thyroid
Body type	Go from gaining weight easily to losing weight	Gradually gain weight which you find extremely hard to lose
Face shape	Face looks drawn, and eyes and cheeks are sunken with dark circles around the eyes	The face is full, round and puffy with bags under the eyes
Facial colouring	Unnaturally pale; sometimes with a grey tinge to the skin	Reddish or rosy-coloured skin
Eyebrows	No change	Hair is sparse and often with the outer one-third to one-half missing
Hair loss	Sometimes	Very common

Body temperature	Fluctuates throughout the day; may wake very hot, then cool, then rise again with extremes in temperature	Steady but low; feel cold much of the time
Best energy time	Extremely tired first thing, as often wake between 2am and 4am then pick up mid-morning; big dip in energy around 4pm then get a second wind	Best in morning having slept, but deteriorates over the day

A simple blood test by your doctor will be able to tell you how well your thyroid is functioning.

Doctors are not always very supportive when it comes to thyroid function. One of the most common medical complaints a doctor hears is feeling tired all the time (commonly referred to as TATT). I am aware of so many people experiencing thyroid symptoms, yet their doctor refuses to acknowledge that this may be the underlying cause of their fatigue. My own doctor told me my results were a fluke, despite my strong family history. If this is your experience, an appointment with a nutritional therapist or dietician could help you.

There's also a simple test that looks at your body temperature. Thyroid hormones affect your metabolic rate, which determines your body temperature. Reduced thyroid function typically manifests as a drop in temperature below the normal. You can easily carry out this test: all you need is a thermometer and a few minutes in the morning before you get out of bed. The test identifies your basal body temperature. It was developed by Dr Broda Barnes MD in the 1940s, and I used it when my doctor refused to acknowledge my hypothyroidism, primarily to reassure myself I was ill and to give me the strength to continue to pester my doctor.

- When should I take the test?
  - For post-menopausal women, take this test for three consecutive mornings at any time.
  - For other women, take the test for three consecutive mornings on days two to four of your cycle.
  - For men, take this test for three consecutive mornings at any time.
  - Do not take the test if you feel you have a cold or sore throat coming or you have had a high amount of alcohol to drink the night before (these can raise your temperature, making the reading invalid).
- What do I do?
  - Keep a thermometer by your bedside. A glass mercury thermometer is the most accurate, but these can be hard to come by (try eBay). You can use a digital thermometer, but be warned that it may be a degree out above or below. Always shake the glass thermometer down after use.
  - As soon as you wake in the morning, put the thermometer under your armpit and lie still for 10 minutes (it is important to move as little as possible). Do not get out of bed until the test is completed.
  - Record the temperature in the chart on the next page.
- What do the results mean?
  - The normal body temperature range is 36.5–36.7°C (97.6–98.2°F).
  - If your temperature was consistently below 36.5°C (97.6°F), this may be an indicator of low metabolic rate and therefore underactive thyroid activity.
  - If your temperature was above 36.7°C (98.2°F), this may be an indicator of high metabolic rate and therefore overactive thyroid activity.

- If the test indicates a high or low reading, consult your doctor.
- If the results are inconsistent, repeat the test again on another day or the next month.

Day	Temperature
1	
2	
3	

6. Boost your microbiome

A healthy microbiome consists of a community of good bacteria, viruses and fungi that live in your digestive tract and perform a variety of functions that are linked to your health and energy. Species such as *lactobacillus* and *bifidobacterium* play an important role in the manufacture of B vitamins and the absorption of nutrients. They help protect you from food sensitivities and promote healthy immune function. They are even linked to having a good night's sleep!

Just like the cells in your body, your microbiome requires food to survive and proliferate. The food that it needs is fibre found in wholegrains and vegetables. The worst thing you can do for your microbiome is to eat a diet high in processed food or low in complex carbohydrates. It starves your good bacteria, allowing the baddies that have been linked to conditions such as irritable bowel syndrome (IBS) to take hold.

Poor thyroid function and chronic stress can also have a significant effect on the health of your microbiome. Low thyroid function slows your metabolic rate, lowering your body temperature and slowing gut mobility. This alters the environment, allowing the baddies, typically yeasts (candida) and bacterium to proliferate, blocking the ability of good bacteria to adhere to the gut wall. In the case of chronic stress, high cortisol levels also slow the peristatic motion of the gut. This slows the movement of food along the tract, allowing the baddies to take hold.

The most natural way to improve the health of your microbiome (and I think the most successful method) is to eat in a way that allows it to thrive. Taking probiotic supplements can help, but they vary in efficacy, so you have no idea how much effect they are having, – this could be an expensive mistake. You should choose a brand carefully (they should always be kept in the fridge), as many brands are a complete waste of money and are destroyed by stomach acid. Symprove is my favourite, and its efficacy is backed up by research at Kings College, University of London.

Here is my advice to improve your microbiome naturally.

- Eat a diet rich in fibre. This means wholegrains such as wheat and oats and a variety of vegetables. Your good bacteria feed on the fibre in these foods, and it's the best way to ensure they colonise. Certain foods – Jerusalem artichoke, chicory root, leeks, onions and asparagus – contain inulin or fructo-oligosaccharide (FOS); these are particularly good food sources for good bacteria.

- Reduce sugar in your diet. Sugar is toxic for your good bacteria and allows the baddies to take over, particularly yeasts such as candida.

- Eat fermented food daily. This could be live unsweetened natural plain yoghurt, kefir (fermented milk drink), tempeh and miso (fermented soybean), sauerkraut (fermented cabbage), kombucha and kimchi pickles. I make my own kefir, and it's so simple. I drink it every day. At lunchtime I have a forkful of sauerkraut – yes, an acquired taste, but I know it's doing me good! You can make sauerkraut or buy it commercially. Just make sure what you buy has not been pasteurised, as this kills the beneficial bacteria.

Part
2

7. Monitor how you eat when feeling stressed

Here is a quick questionnaire. Just tick any that are a "Yes".
- Do you grab food on the run because you have no time to stop and eat?
- Do you avoid breakfast?
- Do you prefer to eat white bread, white rice and white pasta?
- Do you rely on caffeine and sugary foods to keep you going?
- Do you get indigestion?
- Do you suffer from IBS?
- Do you react to certain foods such as gluten or dairy?

If you have answered "Yes" to any of these questions, pay special attention to this section. The chances are stress is affecting your eating and, in the long run, your health.

Stress is managed by your adrenal glands. These are two tiny triangular-shaped glands attached to the top of each of your kidneys. Their function is to produce and secrete a variety of hormones to enable you to deal with trauma, shock and danger – your adrenals are critical for your survival. We know this more commonly as the 'fight or flight' stress response. When we go into 'fight or flight', these hormones command various organs and tissues in your body to prepare themselves to either fight the stressor or flee from it. This boosts your energy and your capacity to cope when faced with sudden or heightened pressure, challenges and trauma.

This is why chronic stress alters your food-eating habits! You need a quick surge of energy, and the quickest way to get that is from simple carbohydrates and stimulants. It's not such a problem if this happens fairly infrequently, but that's no longer the case in this crazy, highly demanding world we now live in. So many of us are stuck in 'fight or flight' and find it hard to switch off. Your brain cannot distinguish between what is a genuine life-threatening danger and what is only a bit of pressure that will pass. Chronic stress puts you on the blood sugar rollercoaster (see earlier); and, to compound this further, if your sleep is disrupted, the effects will be even worse (more on this in Chapter 4).

As well as stress putting you on the blood sugar rollercoaster, it will also increase your demand for certain nutrients. Your adrenal glands will be using up vitamin C like there's no tomorrow. The changes in your physiology caused by cortisol flooding your system will trigger pain and inflammation – which also increases your demand for nutrients. Your thyroid gland will be struggling to cope, and your pancreas will be feeling the pressure of having to release more and more insulin. This has the potential to upset the balance of your endocrine system and in the long run, rather than energise you for survival, will actually exhaust you. You could even burn out, and that's no fun at all. You'll have no energy, you'll feel demotivated and despondent, even depressed, and you won't have the energy to get yourself out of it alone.

As stress impacts your digestive system, you may notice you're becoming sensitive to certain food types. Gluten, dairy, soya, citrus fruits? I was a dinner party nightmare when I was burning out. One minute I couldn't tolerate wheat. The next, yeast. Then soya (which is in so many processed foods). Then nuts. It was miserable and I had to take back control of my eating. Now I'm fine.

As well as eating a varied, healthy diet, you should also ensure you take sufficient time to eat. Stress lowers the amount of acid in your stomach, which makes it hard to digest proteins. Take time to eat. If you want to absorb nutrients from your food, you need to give it time. Whatever you do, don't bolt your food down on the run. Calm, mindful eating that allows your digestive system to do its job and not be influenced by stress hormones, is the best way to help your body digest food. Focus on your food. Be mindful of what you are eating, not the problem you have at work that you need to rush back to.

Here are some ideas for an adrenal-friendly kitchen.

Nutrient	Food source
Vitamin B: Needed to produce cortisol and maintain energy levels, particularly B5. B vitamins include: • B1 (thiamine) • B2 (riboflavin) • B3 (Niacin) • B5 (Pantothenic acid) • B6, Folates, Biotin	Wholegrains – wholewheat, wheatgerm, rye, barley, oats, brown rice, wild rice Green leafy vegetables – greens, kale, spinach, Brussels sprouts, broccoli Mushrooms Eggs – free range Nuts – almonds, Brazil nuts, walnuts (unsalted and not heat-treated) Seeds – sunflower, pumpkin, sesame, hemp, chia, flax (all unsalted and not heat-treated)
Vitamin C: Supports adrenal gland function, the production of cortisol adrenal recovery. Stress increases the excretion of vitamin C	Citrus fruit – orange, grapefruit and lemon but not neat fruit juices Berries – blackberries, blueberries, raspberries, strawberries Other fruit – kiwi fruit Salad – red and green peppers, watercress, tomatoes Vegetables – broccoli, peas, sweet potato, pumpkin, vegetable juices such as V8
Minerals – calcium and magnesium: Help to relax and calm the mind and body	Magnesium: green leafy vegetables (broccoli, cabbage, kale, spinach), almonds, Brazil nuts, pumpkin seeds, sesame seeds and pineapple Calcium: dairy products, spinach, seeds, sardines
Good fats (Omega 3, 6 and 9): Help support immunity and reduce inflammation caused by stress	Oily fish – salmon, trout, mackerel, fresh tuna (not tinned) Nuts – almonds, Brazil nuts, walnuts (all unsalted and not heat-treated)

	Seeds – sunflower, pumpkin, sesame, hemp, chia, flax (all unsalted and not heat-treated) Eggs – high-omega-fed eggs Avocado Oils: extra virgin olive, hemp, walnut, coconut Nut butter – cashew, almond
Theanine: Helps you relax by increasing alpha waves in the brain	All tea without milk, but particularly green tea
Water: To keep the body and mind hydrated and functioning	Water – about eight glasses of water a day or 1.5 litres. Herbal and fruit teas – chamomile, liquorice and passionflower

Activities to learn more about how far nutrition optimises your energy

Part
2

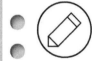

Activity 1: Your energy audit: energy boosters and drainers

Different foods affect blood sugar levels to different degrees. How is your diet affecting your blood sugar levels?

1. Think about what you ate yesterday.
2. Go systematically through the next chart and record in the Tally boxes how many times you would have eaten these foods.
3. Add up each column and see whether your overall diet was boosting or draining your energy.

Sustainable fuel	Tally	Rocket fuel	Tally
Wholemeal sliced bread, pitta, rolls		White sliced bread, rolls, baguettes	
Rye bread		Croissants, bagels, crumpets	
Oatcakes		Cheese crackers	
Porridge		White rice cakes	
Wholewheat pasta		Breakfast cereals	
Brown rice		Cakes, pastries, doughnuts, scones, waffles	
Brown basmati rice		Sweets, biscuits, cookies, chocolate bars	
Wholegrains (quinoa, buckwheat, bulgur wheat – when cooked al dente)		Crisps, popcorn	
Green leafy vegetables (kale, spinach, broccoli, courgette, green beans)		White, corn and rice pasta	
White vegetables (cauliflower, cabbage, radishes)		White rice	
Mushrooms		Pizza	
Salad (lettuce, cucumber, rocket, watercress, peppers, tomatoes)		Vegetables (potatoes, parsnips, swedes)	
Fruit (berries, cherries, plums, apples, pears, oranges, grapefruit)		Chips, mashed potato	
Pulses (lentil, chickpeas, beans)		Low-fat processed foods such as low-fat mayonnaise	
Lean meat		Fruit (over-ripe bananas, grapes, pineapple)	

Sustainable fuel	Tally	Rocket fuel	Tally
Fish		Dried fruits (apricots, cranberries, dates, figs, sultanas)	
Eggs		Fruit-flavoured yoghurt	
Cheese		Tinned fruit in sugar syrup	
Nuts (almonds, Brazils, walnuts)		Jam, jelly	
Seeds (pumpkin, sunflower, sesame, chia, linseed/flax, hemp)		Puddings such as mousse, fruit pies	
Plain yoghurt		Table sugar	
Tea (redbush, herbal and fruit teas)		Ice cream	
Water		Fruit squash, fruit juices, smoothies	
		Tea, coffee	
		Hot chocolate	
		Fizzy drinks (cola, lemonade)	
		Energy drinks (such as Lucozade, Red Bull)	
		Alcohol	
Total		**Total**	

Part
2

The blood sugar rollercoaster can have an enormous effect on our energy, mood and productivity. If you experience extreme highs and lows in energy during the day and eventually an energy slump, complete the next exercise.

Activity 2: The blood sugar rollercoaster

Take some time to consider how you feel at different times of the day and what you have eaten.

1. Record your answers on the chart below:

Part 2

Period	How did I feel?	What did I eat during this period?
Early morning		
Mid-morning		
Lunchtime		
Mid-afternoon		
Early evening		
Evening		

Are you feeling this way because you are hyper and buzzing, or low and craving? Give the strength of this feeling a score. For example, if you feel you're buzzing or agitated, then if this feeling is very strong, score a 5; if it's weak, score a 1. If you feel faint and weak or maybe you're craving something sweet, how strong is this feeling? Score −5 if it is very strong and −1 if it is a weak symptom.

2. Put an X in the square on the chart below that represents your scores, to create a rough illustration of your personal blood sugar rollercoaster.

Part

2

Score	Early morning	Mid-morning	Lunchtime	Mid-afternoon	Early evening	Evening
5						
4						
3						
2						
1						
Balanced						
−1						
−2						
−3						
−4						
−5						

3. Before you identify some changes you can make, ask yourself the following and record your answers in the right-hand column:

Ask yourself	Your answer
How many times a week do you skip breakfast?	
What is your typical breakfast?	
How many glasses of water do you drink each day?	
What are you most likely to drink as a pick-me-up?	
What are you most likely to snack on?	
How often do you eat carb-rich foods at lunchtime?	
What types of bread, rice and pasta do you eat?	
How many days a week do you eat five servings of fruit and veg?	
How many times a week do you eat oily fish such as salmon, herring and mackerel?	

Part 2

4. Review the 'stop and replace' chart opposite. Place a tick in the column by the foods you feel able to change.

Stop or reduce...	✓	Replace with...
Branded cereals such as cornflakes or puffed rice		Porridge, home-made sugar-free muesli, shredded wheat, or natural live yoghurt and some berries
White toast and jam/honey/marmalade		Boiled egg and wholemeal toast
White bread sandwich, roll or baguette		Sandwich using wholemeal bread/pitta/wrap or rye bread
Baked or mashed potato		Brown or basmati rice, mashed sweet potato
Sugary snacks – crisps, biscuits, popcorn, chocolate bars, pretzels		Small handful of nuts or seeds, some vegetable sticks with hummus or guacamole, or a piece of fruit
Rice cakes or cheese crackers		Oatcakes
Fruit yoghurt		Plain yoghurt and frozen berries
Cola, lemonade, energy drink		Fizzy water with lemon or lime juice squeezed in
Coffee, strong tea or hot chocolate		Coffee alternative, fruit or herb tea, or water

Part

2

5. What changes are you going to make to your diet to balance your blood sugar and prevent the blood sugar rollercoaster?

Stop eating/drinking!	Start eating/drinking!

To remain motivated, make small, gradual changes to your diet. Choose one change per week, or only change once you are comfortable with your previous change. If you are reducing caffeinated drinks, reduce consumption gradually over a period of two weeks.

If your diet is quite varied, it may help you to complete a three-day food diary and review what you have eaten over that period.

Activity 3: Your three-day food diary
The energy audit exercise just looked at one day, but it's often more helpful to review what you have eaten over a three-day period.

1. To do this you will need to make a record of everything you eat and drink. Use the chart below.

Be honest, because this will help you identify why you may feel low in energy. It may be that you are not eating enough.

	Breakfast	Lunch	Dinner	Snacks
Day 1	Time: What I ate:	Time: What I ate:	Time: What I ate:	Time: What I ate:

Day 2	Time: What I ate:	Time: What I ate:	Time: What I ate:	Time: What I ate:
Day 3	Time: What I ate:	Time: What I ate:	Time: What I ate:	Time: What I ate:

Part
2

2. Look at the chart on the next page to get some ideas on what you can eat each day that will provide you with energy and nutrients and balance your blood sugar.

Breakfast ideas	Lunch ideas	Dinner ideas	Snack ideas
• Porridge with berries or grated apples and ground seeds • Sugar-free muesli with nuts and seeds and cinnamon • Unsweetened yoghurt and berries • Boiled or poached egg with wholewheat toast or mushrooms • Poached egg with spinach • Scrambled egg and smoked salmon • French toast made with wholewheat bread • Hard-boiled egg and Parma ham • NutriBullet smoothie with added flax seeds and chia seeds for protein • Protein shake	• Greek salad • Salad niçoise • Tomato, mozzarella and avocado salad • Mackerel, horseradish and beetroot salad • Omelette/ frittata with Parma ham and mushrooms or red peppers • Wrap with chicken, fish or hummus and salad • Food from previous evening's meal • Brown rice or quinoa or can of lentils with mixed chopped peppers, tomato, cucumber, beetroot and feta cheese • Home-made soup with meat and lentils • Tinned salmon and cucumber open sandwich made with one slice of bread	• Chicken or pork casserole with onions, carrots, celery • Roast meat and roast or mashed sweet potatoes and green leafy vegetables • Chicken and noodle stir fry • Cottage pie with sweet potato topping • Lamb chop with roast sweet potatoes and salsa verde • Home-made meat or vegetarian curry with wild rice • Salmon en papillote with chopped celery and tarragon and asparagus, new potatoes • Baked cod on lentils and peppers • Lentil and chickpea curry • Stuffed red peppers	• Few unsalted nuts • Small palm-full of seeds • Oatcake with hummus or nut butter • Ryvita and cottage cheese • Oatcake with cheese • Half wholewheat pitta bread and mackerel pâté • Small piece of cheese and an apple • Small plain yoghurt and fruit • Carrot and celery sticks with hummus or guacamole • Celery and nut butter • Hard-boiled egg • Cold meat – chicken • Roll of smoked salmon • Protein shake made with coconut milk

Stimulants boost your energy when you're flagging because they trigger the stress response which instructs the liver to release some of its stored glucose into the bloodstream, thereby raising your low blood sugar. They'll also give you a lift for about an hour by triggering dopamine in your brain, which satisfies your need for a reward.

Activity 4: Are you addicted to stimulants?

1. Look at the stimulants listed in the left-hand column of the table below and record the number of times you used each stimulant during the course of a day.
2. Add up the total number of units. If your energy levels are good, you are allowed 2–3 units before it would have a detrimental effect. If you experience low energy and you want to improve your energy, your score needs to be zero until you feel your energy improve. Look at the right-hand column and determine what you can do to lower your stimulant score.

Part 2

Stimulant – per unit	Tally of units per day	Alternative
Caffeine:		**Tea:**
• Tea – 1 cup		• Reduce the strength or use a smaller mug
• Espresso – half shot		• Try redbush tea, herb or fruit tea
• Americano – 1 cup		**Coffee:**
• Green tea – 2 cups		• Reduce by one cup per day per week
• Cola – 1 cup		• Try Barleycup, Yannoh, Caro or dandelion coffee as an alternative
• Red Bull – 1 can		
• Caffeine pills – 1 pill		
• Dark chocolate – 70g		
• Milk chocolate – 200g		

		Energy drinks (cola, Red Bull, Lucozade): • Gradually reduce until you have cut out **Chocolate** (bars or drink): • Replace with carob snacks or drinks
Sugar: • In hot drink – 1 teaspoon • Cake – per half-portion • Biscuit – per portion • Sweets – per sweet • Hidden in foods – per 5g		• Gradually cut back the amount you add to hot drinks, one teaspoon each week • Replace sugary cereals with suggestions in the menu chart • Avoid dried fruits – have a piece of fruit instead • Dilute fruit juice, then give up • Check labels for added sugar • Avoid sugar substitutes
Alcohol: • Beer, lager, cider – per half-pint • Wine – per 80ml glass • Spirits – per 25ml measure • Mixers – per mixer		• Ideally have an alcohol-free month while you're rebuilding your energy Otherwise: • Have alcohol-free days during the week • Cut out drinking at lunchtime • Set yourself a weekly goal of the maximum number of units • Drink a glass of water after each alcoholic drink, to reduce overall consumption
Cigarettes: Per cigarette, cigar		• Get support to reduce from your doctor or local hospital
Total units per day		

What can I do to lower my score?	When will I do this?

Your reflections

What has resonated with you while reading Step 1: Nutrition for optimum energy?

- What have you learned about yourself?
- What have you learned about your nutritional intake and absorption?
- What have you learned about how nutrition may be the reason for your low energy?
- What do you need to start doing that you have not done before?
- What other thoughts do you have?

Part
2

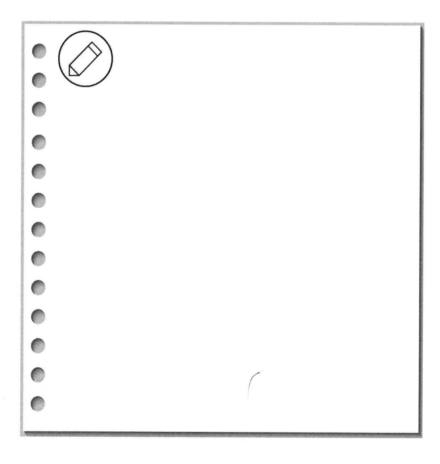

CHAPTER 5

Step 2: Sleep for optimum energy

◊ Does it take you longer than twenty minutes to fall asleep?
◊ Do you wake abruptly in the night and find that your whole to-do list flashes into your mind?
◊ Do you regularly experience disturbed sleep?
◊ Do you need an alarm to wake you up at the right time?
◊ Do you still feel unrefreshed and groggy when you get up?
◊ Do you find yourself becoming sleepy during the day?
◊ Do you work shifts?

If you've answered "Yes" to any of these questions, pay extra special attention to this section.

Sleep is a big issue. It's essential for energy, yet so many people complain about how little sleep they get, or how disturbed their sleep is. Next to the weather, it's probably the next most talked-about subject!

It's also a topic of great frustration. I hear it so often: "If only I didn't have to sleep; it seems such a waste of time." But it's not. We know it makes us feel good and gives us the energy to get through the day. Sleep is all about rest, restoration and repair, and it's vital if we want to be able to think clearly, concentrate, deliver effectively, interact well and appreciate those around us. Our bodies have evolved to be very busy while we sleep.

- We release growth hormones to help us grow muscle and repair the damage caused to the body during the day.
- Our liver detoxes toxins.
- Our mind processes the emotions we've built up during the day by dreaming through the use of metaphor and imagery.
- We consolidate and embed our daily memories from short-term to long-term memory.
- The cerebral spinal fluid that surrounds our brain and spinal cord clears the by-products from the brain cells' activity that day.

Getting through all these activities effectively means that we should be working to develop a consistent sleep pattern.

Your night-time sleeping is programmed to follow a particular pattern of ninety-minute cycles, although these can differ depending on age. Initially you move between wakefulness and sleep referred to as *NREM1 (non-rapid eye movement 1)*, as slower alpha and theta waves take over from the day's excitable beta waves that keep you alert. Stage 2 follows, *NREM2*, where your temperature drops and your brain produces slower, calmer alpha waves. You now drift into sleep, albeit lightly – you could easily awaken. Stage 3 happens next, *NREM3*, and is the start of a deeper, restorative sleep, signified by slow delta waves. You will be less responsive to your environment. This is the time when various hormones, including growth hormone, are released to repair muscles and soft tissue and your immune system rebalances. Finally, Stage 4, *rapid eye movement* sleep (*REM*), is where you sleep deeply but your mind becomes very active and your eyes move rapidly. This is the stage where you dream, processing the information from the day, and lay down long-term memories.

Part
2

During a good night's sleep, you will repeat these cycles five or six times. It is following this pattern without interruption that will leave you refreshed. As you move from one cycle to another and from deep sleep to a lighter sleep, you may stir, but this is only momentary and does not tend to disturb you.

It takes the average 'healthy sleeper' twenty minutes to fall asleep. Falling asleep at 11pm and following five cycles has the potential to have you waking refreshed at 6.30am. On top of this, your first two cycles of sleep are the most restorative. This means you should not be picking and choosing how long you sleep for each night depending on what's going on in the social calendar or how much extra work you need to do at home to keep on top of work demands. It also means that building up a sleep deficit during the week and then sleeping for a whole day at the weekend will do nothing to help your energy or your health. This is because an irregular sleep pattern plays havoc with your natural circadian rhythm. This is your body's physical, mental and behavioural changes over a twenty-four-hour period, typically referred to as your 'body clock'. Messed-up sleep means a messed-up body clock. Finding a way to achieve a regular sleep pattern is the priority.

Although, individually, we all need differing amounts of sleep, an abundance of research tells us that the optimum amount for health is seven to eight hours; this is also the guideline from the World Health Organisation. Too little and also too much have consequences to how well you mentally function (cognitive ability).

Yet 30 per cent of us have trouble getting off to sleep, and an astonishing 85 per cent wake feeling unrefreshed. This doesn't surprise me when we're living chaotic lives, surviving on refined food, stimulants and stress hormones, all of which have a significant effect on our sleep patterns and subsequent energy and health.

Not only does a lack of sleep create dark bags under your eyes – it also affects the activity of many of your genes plus your physical and mental processes. There is an abundance of research out there demonstrating that a lack of sleep has been connected to health conditions such as cardiovascular disease, diabetes, obesity and Alzheimer's disease. Why? Well, firstly it activates the stress response triggering the release of adrenalin and cortisol, which alter the body's physiology as part of the 'fight or flight' response.

A lack of sleep or broken sleep cycles will also leave you feeling drowsy, forgetful and unfocused, as energy levels in the brain have not been restored during the night. You may crave quick energy foods, because sleep controls the appetite hormone *ghrelin*; so less sleep means you want to eat more, and in the long term the impact on your immune system can affect your health. Amnesty International lists sleep deprivation as a form of torture!

You know you've had a good night's sleep when you wake feeling refreshed in the morning and haven't needed the alarm clock. If this isn't the case, it's time to take stock and identify the root cause. Is it feeling chronically stressed, niggling worries, too much noise in the street – or maybe light in the bedroom, or even the blue light from using laptops and smartphones until you go to bed? If you're overweight and a heavy snorer and suspect you suffer from sleep apnoea, where your throat blocks your breathing momentarily while you sleep, you need to seek medical advice.

Waking and sleeping at the same times each day is a great way to reset your circadian rhythms, which control alertness during the day. Getting quality rest each night leads to more energy in the mornings.

1.   Create a bedtime routine

Our bodies love routine, so creating a consistent bedtime routine is one of the most important things you can do. This means going to bed and getting up at the same times every day. By doing this, your internal clock will be primed to trigger the pineal gland in your brain to release the sleep hormone, *melatonin*, at a specific time. Providing you have an evening routine that allows for some relaxation, your body will be routinely preparing you for sleep and you will be much more likely to sleep soundly.

Choose a time to fall asleep that allows you to achieve five to six sleep cycles. This means if you want to wake at 7am, you need to be asleep by 11.30pm, which means going to bed at 11pm. Your genes will determine whether you're a morning or night person and even how long it takes you to get to sleep, so you will need to take this into account. My advice, though, is to always set a routine that allows you to get some sleep before midnight. This will allow your body clock to trigger the release of human growth hormone, which is required for your body to repair.

It may take some time to create this routine. There is little point in going to bed at 10pm if you feel wide awake and know you will be lying there for a considerable time. All this will do is generate anxiety, and you will obsess about not being able to sleep, which makes it even less likely that sleep will happen.

I am always a bit wary of using sleep apps on your phone that monitor how you've slept that night. Firstly, the apps are not particularly accurate and make you anxious about the amount of sleep you're getting, which perpetuates the problem. Secondly, it is not a good idea to have your phone by your bedside. Alerts and messages have the potential to wake you, and the electromagnetic waves released by phones can disturb sleep patterns. You're better off leaving your phone charging in the kitchen.

If you do wake in the night, here are some tips to get back to sleep:

- Do not look at the clock during the night. This will only panic you and make you even more awake.
- As soon as you wake, do not allow yourself to think of anything other than your breathing. Focus on your in-breath and your out-breath. Count to four, hold for two, then breathe out for four.

Part
2

- Forget counting sheep – it requires too much concentration. If breathing hasn't worked for you, try a body scan meditation where you focus on different parts of the body, tensing then relaxing each in turn, beginning at the feet and working up to the head.
- Waking in the night can often be down to low blood sugar. If this is the case for you, a small snack before bed may help you.
- If all fails, get out of bed and go into another room. Do not put too much light on and definitely do not look at your phone or turn on the television.

Do not go to bed early the next night if you didn't sleep well the previous night. It will upset your pattern. If disturbed sleep goes on for a few nights, then it is actually better to try going to bed later, which will make your sleep more efficient; and do not spend longer in bed, which would put pressure on you to try to go to sleep.

If this is a problem, I would advise some sleep training. You will initially be limiting your sleep to five hours. This might sound contradictory to what I have been saying about needing seven to eight hours' sleep, but bear with me. Rather than spending eight hours in bed tossing and turning and worrying about not getting enough sleep, this will drive your brain to achieve deeper sleep and set a new sleep pattern. Then, over a period of time, you can bring the time you go to sleep forward until you find a time that works for you.

Although seven to eight hours is optimal, it is more about quality than quantity. Start by working out when you want to wake up. Let's say that is 7am. A five-hour sleep means going to sleep at 2am. You are not allowed to take any naps in the day or evening before this, and you must wake up and get up when the alarm goes off (no hitting the snooze button). Your mind will soon realise that the short time it has for sleep needs to be used efficiently… and it is. You will sleep more deeply and continuously.

If you go to sleep later at the weekend or on a day off from work, this does not mean you can sleep in. You still need to wake at the same time the next day, or certainly no more than thirty minutes later.

I am cautious about being too prescriptive about daytime napping, as the research is so mixed on this topic and taking a nap in the day is very much a personal thing. What I will say, though, is that it's all about routine and setting your body clock. Our ancestors would have gone to bed when it got dark. During the long winter months, they would have woken at some stage during the night to eat or for sex, then gone back to sleep again. They set their body clocks that way. Many cultures have a siesta in the afternoon, eat later and go to bed later. Sleep is counted over a twenty-four-hour period rather than one fixed block of time. For me, if I take a nap it completely messes up my sleep; for others it's an imperative.

What I will be prescriptive about, though, is that napping on the sofa in the evening is a definite no-no. If you are doing this, you haven't taken the opportunities during the day to recharge your batteries. Spending five or ten minutes sitting in a chair, taking some deep breaths, allows the mind to calm and recharge you for the rest of the day.

Part 2

How you wake up in the morning will have a big impact on how positive, motivated and energised you feel. Here are some ideas:

- Use a dawn simulation alarm clock, which slowly lightens the room.
- Set your alarm clock to play your favourite music station.
- Place your alarm clock away from your bed – so you have to get out of bed to turn it off.
- Make the first thought that pops into your mind in the morning an energising one.
- Do some stretching exercises to get your blood flowing.

2.   Make your bedroom sleep-friendly

There's this funny term, 'sleep hygiene', which I think sounds as if your sleep has to be clean but actually means good sleep habits! If you want a good night's sleep, this is what you need to be doing.

- Have a comfortable bed. Change your mattress every seven years.
- Make sure your bedroom is cool. You are more likely to fall asleep when your body is cool, so turn down the heating in your bedroom. Studies show the best temperature is between 16°C and 18°C.
- Make sure your bedroom is as quiet as you can make it, and dark. If you live near a busy road or have noisy neighbours, wear ear plugs. A blackout blind on the window or an eye shield will keep the light out.
- Turn your alarm clock away – so the light does not bother you, and to prevent you looking at it should you wake in the night.
- Do not have a television in your bedroom. The blue light suppresses the release of the sleep hormone, melatonin. A television is also telling your brain you need to remain alert, even when it is switched off.
- Do not work in your bedroom.

3.   Eat right to sleep well

What you consume has a profound effect on how well you sleep.

Top of the list to avoid are caffeine and alcohol. Caffeine in coffee, tea and cola drinks, even dark chocolate, should be avoided after 4pm. They alter your blood sugar balance, which stimulates the release of cortisol.

Alcohol is a sedative that you may think calms you, but it actually disrupts the rapid eye movement part of your sleep cycle, prohibiting the restorative benefits of sleep. Like caffeine, it disrupts your blood sugar balance, and disrupts the storage of glycogen (glucose) in the liver, so you struggle to maintain your blood glucose levels during the night, and so you wake up.

A heavy meal two hours before bedtime will disrupt your sleep. If you do need to eat late, try to avoid heavy meat and rich sauces, which require more digestion.

Some foods can assist sleep because they are high in the amino acid *tryptophan*, which is converted in the brain to serotonin and then into melatonin, the sleep hormone. If you struggle to go to sleep or to remain asleep, then just before you go to bed have a warm milky drink or some chicken, turkey or cottage cheese on an oatcake, or a banana or two kiwi fruit. These can be particularly useful if you're waking in the night hungry.

I have found drinking sour cherry juice helpful, because it contains melatonin. A small cup of camomile tea is calming on the mind (not too big or you'll be waking in the night to visit the toilet).

Taking a supplement called *5-HTP* can be helpful. This is converted by the body into serotonin (the good mood hormone), then melatonin (the sleep hormone). Do *not* take it if you are on any antidepressant or anti-anxiety medication, as these are already working on the serotonin balance in your brain.

Recent research has been flagging up the link between the gut microbiome (good bacteria in the gut) and insomnia. The good bacteria in the gut feed on indigestible plant fibre in foods such as leeks, onions, Jerusalem artichoke, garlic, asparagus and bananas. These are referred to as *prebiotics*, which promote the growth of healthy bacteria. You can incorporate more of these foods in your diet, but what I have found best is to have a prebiotic drink just before bedtime.

Prem's story

Prem found it really difficult to fall asleep each night. It had got to the stage where he dreaded going to bed as he knew he would just lie there, with an active mind and no hope of sleep.

This wasn't something new. He'd been like this since his teenage years, but it was getting worse. He'd taken sleeping tablets for a short time, but hated the way they made him feel groggy the next day, and after about six months he stopped.

When Prem came to see me and we chatted about his sleep patterns, I noticed that it appeared worse in the winter months. Prem agreed with this and confirmed that his mood also dropped during the winter. While he never felt the need to see a doctor about this, he described it as "feeling fed up" but still coping, even if he was miserable.

Prem's difficulty falling asleep and his low mood suggested to me that there was a chance his serotonin levels were low. A urine test confirmed this. I recommended some changes to Prem's diet that involved increasing his protein intake, which was very low, and I suggested he took a daily morning walk during daylight hours. Both of these can help to increase serotonin. Serotonin is converted to melatonin, the sleep hormone, once darkness falls. Prem needed a bit of extra help to improve his serotonin. I suggested a supplement of 5-HTP, a compound which, as mentioned above, is converted into serotonin.

As a result, Prem's sleep patterns started to improve significantly and, although they were not perfect, he no longer worried about going to bed.

4.   Banish worry and anxiety

The levels of stress and anxiety are escalating. Health insurers' online counselling services are finding that anxiety is becoming the primary reason for contacting them. Anxiety is the principal cause of difficulty in falling asleep and staying asleep.

Worry and anxiety trigger cortisol, the stress hormone. Issues get talked over and over in the mind; scenarios are generated that may never happen in real life, yet seem so real and plausible in your head. The sheer amount of activity can use so much energy. The signs can be that you are struggling to get to sleep as you cannot switch your mind off, or you may be waking abruptly during the night. You may find you're grinding your teeth or clenching your jaw, or you have a headache or tension in your neck and shoulders that you cannot clear.

Whatever may be the symptom, if you are going to get to sleep and sleep soundly, you need to ensure that the levels of cortisol – the hormone triggered when you worry, which keeps you alert to solve the problem – is reduced to a low level. This will only happen when you learn to switch off worry and anxiety.

Taking part in some exercise is good and helps you switch off from the worries built up over the day, but avoid high-intensity exercise two hours before you retire for bed. If going out and exercising isn't your thing, any activity that distracts you enough to switch off the internal chatter is good for reducing anxiety. This could be reading a good book, or absorbing yourself in music, doing a craft or some gardening. It is your choice and very individual, but it must be something that completely distracts you.

Keeping a worry diary can help you to identify what your worries are, what the root cause is and what you can do about the problem that's triggering you to worry. I have an example of a worry diary in the activities below. It's then over to you to take action.

Another helpful tip is to keep a pad and pencil by your bed and write down your thoughts and worries before you go to sleep. This way, you are offloading them from your mind. You can also do this if you wake worrying during the night. Follow this by taking some time to reflect on the positive things that have happened that day. Relive and re-savour these happy memories.

5.   Take control of your technology

We have become addicted to our phones, tablets and computers. All these different social media apps have us clutching our phones until the very minute we go to bed. They are an absolute sleep saboteur, a menace of the first degree, and I have to admit that if I am not strict with myself I can be just as bad.

Firstly, they keep the beta waves in the brain activated, so you remain alert and engaged when you should be calming the mind and preparing for sleep. Every time we post something or respond to an alert, we release dopamine – the chemical that provides us with a sense of reward and motivation – in the brain. It's what makes emails and social media so addictive. We've become so addicted to being 'always on', we start to withdraw when the mind is calming in the evening, making us even more likely to reach for the phone and get a fix of dopamine. It's giving us a positive feedback and we feel awake, buzzing and energised.

Secondly, the bluish light emitted from the screens blocks the release of melatonin for around ninety minutes. If you want to sleep well, you have to switch off your digital devices in plenty of time before bed. I call this an 'electronic sundown', and ideally, if you want to sleep well and feel refreshed the next day, you need to turn off your computer, tablet and smartphone at least ninety minutes before bed. This means *no* emails and social media after this time. For the same reason, do not have a TV in your bedroom or charge your mobile devices in your bedroom.

6. Follow practices to calm your mind

Living this 'always-on' life means we have to actively make ourselves relax and switch off. If you want to sleep well and allow melatonin to do its job, you need to create calming evening rituals that allow your mind to switch off from the craziness of the day around two hours before bed.

This means no emailing or work activities!

Here are some ideas:

- Try mindfulness meditation or deep breathing just before bedtime. It activates the slower, calmer alpha waves, which signals to the brain that we are relaxing. Studies are finding that it halves the time it takes to fall asleep by reducing cortisol levels. It helps you to live in the moment and reduce worry and anxiety caused by the past or the future.

- Light a fragrant candle and have a warm, relaxing bath two hours before bedtime. Add some lavender oil – or some Epsom salts, which contain magnesium, which relaxes muscles. As your body cools, it will make you feel sleepy just about the time you go to bed. Chinese medicine views a warm bath as an opportunity to balance the flow of life energy, called *qi*.

- Try some natural herb extracts of valerian root or passionflower extract, which have a calming, sedative effect on the mind. You can also take some if you wake in the night.

- Have a massage to relax muscles and calm you.

- Download tracks of pink noise from YouTube and play while sleeping. Pink noise contains a mix of balanced sounds at high and low frequencies within our hearing range that calm the mind by slowing brain waves.

- Keep the lights low in the room you are sitting in one hour before retiring for bed.

- Keep a gratitude diary. Before you settle to sleep, record three

Part
2

things in your diary you are grateful for that day. This helps your mind to feel more positive about your day and reduces elevated stress hormones.

- Spray your pillow with a sleep spray. They contain calming, relaxing essential oils.

7. Get a dose of morning sunlight

The vital sleep hormone, melatonin, is produced from the conversion of the happy hormone, serotonin. Serotonin is triggered by sunlight and melatonin by darkness. It is why getting out in the sunshine makes you feel so good and why gloomy, dreary winter days have been associated with a mild depression called *seasonal affective disorder* (*SAD*).

Part
2

Getting thirty minutes of daylight, particularly if you spend your day shut up in an artificially lit workplace, not only starts the process of producing melatonin rolling but also helps to reset your natural body clock's sleep-wake cycle. This means that you feel awake and energised during the day, and, providing you don't hit the social media app on your phone, calm and relaxed and ready to sleep for the night in the evening. Even dull days have an effect!

So… get off the bus a few stops earlier, or park your car as far from the office as feasible.

Activities to learn more about how far sleep optimises your energy

Sleep isn't something that just happens. You have to plan for it by creating the right environment and following certain practices. Use the next exercise to identify the quality of your sleep and what may be causing you to experience problems.

Activity 1: What is the quality of your sleep?
1. If you're not getting seven to eight hours' sleep, keep a three-night sleep diary to identify your sleep pattern.
2. Record your sleep habits in the chart below.

	Night 1	Night 2	Night 3
How many hours did I sleep for in total?			
What did I do during the evening – eat, drink, exercise?			
How would I rate my levels of stress and anxiety during the day?			
What time did I get into bed?			
How long did it take to fall asleep?			
Did I sleep through the night?			
What times do I think I woke during the night?			
How long was I awake for?			
What was on my mind?			
How did I wake up in the morning – naturally or by the alarm clock?			
How did I feel on waking?			
Did I use anything to 'get me going'?			
Did I catch up on sleep during the day?			

Activity 2: Your worry diary

Worry absorbs our minds, distracts us and saps our energy. To avoid using too much energy, you need to identify just how important that worry is and what the solution is.

1. List all your worries and their sources below. The source can be work, family, friends, major life events, financial worries or health concerns.
2. Score each worry between 1 and 10 according to how significant it is, where 1 is not very significant and 10 is extremely worrying.
3. Ask yourself how much control you have over solving each worry. Tick the worries that you have some control over solving.

Part 2

Worry	Source	Score	✓

4. Worrying about something does not solve it. Identify a maximum of three worries that are the most important to you right now, and write them down in the table below.
5. What actions can you take to solve them or at least reduce the severity of the worry? Consider what you will need to do, and who else you can involve to help with this or at least support you.

Three worries I have control over	Action I can take now

Activity 3: What action can you take to improve your sleep?

From what you have read so far in this chapter, what could you do to improve your sleep cycle? Consider the seven ways and identify three remedies:

1. Create a bedtime routine
2. Make your bedroom sleep-friendly
3. Eat right to sleep well
4. Banish worry and anxiety
5. Take control of your technology
6. Follow practices to calm your mind
7. Get a dose of morning sunlight

Part 2

Three remedies:
1.
2.
3.

Activity 4: Your to-do list

To clear your mind of the thoughts about what you need to do the next day, it helps to write them down, using a chart based on the one below. This can calm the mind, which aids your sleep.

1. At the end of each day, identify everything you need to do the next day and write it down.
2. Then ask yourself: is it important to do tomorrow; can it wait for another day; if so, when; and finally do I really need to do it at all?
3. When tomorrow comes, start with the activity that is most important and will give you the greatest sense of achievement. This will energise and motivate you for the day. Try to avoid starting with emails. These will divert your attention and drain your energy.

Part 2

Activity	I will do it tomorrow	I will do it another time – when? Record it in your diary	I will never do it

Your reflections

What has resonated with you while reading Step 2: Sleep for optimum energy?

- What have you learned about yourself?
- What have you learned about the state of your sleep cycle?
- What have you learned about how sleep may be the reason for your low energy?
- What do you need to start doing that you have not done before?
- What other thoughts do you have?

CHAPTER 6

Step 3: Movement for optimum energy

◊ Do you avoid exercise because you feel too tired?
◊ Do you find it too difficult to find the time to exercise?
◊ Do you frequently make excuses for not exercising?
◊ Do you hate the gym but not know what else to do?
◊ Do you spend most of your day sitting at your desk?
◊ Do you have a long commute which leaves you sitting down?
◊ Do you have an injury that is preventing you from exercising?

If you've answered "Yes" to any of these questions, pay extra special attention to this section.

It's likely that movement, or to be more precise, the lack of it, may be contributing to your low energy, and you need to develop a regime that gets your body off a chair, onto your feet and into action.

Lives have become more sedentary with sitting for the long commute to work, sitting at a desk all day in front of a screen, then going home and sitting in a different chair in front of another screen. It's little wonder you feel depleted of energy. You could be sitting for at least ten hours a day, most days.

It's a Catch 22. Exercise energises us, but we also need energy to exercise. Add to that, that too much exercise requiring physical strength and endurance could be depleting you of energy. Getting the right amount of exercise plays a big part in the whole energy conversation.

As we cram so much into our daily lives, many of us now find it hard to find the time to fit exercise in… and even if we do, it's the first to go when something crops up.

Exercise is powerful! The rise in oxygen and the production of hormones such as endorphins, serotonin and dopamine have a positive effect on our mind, body, moods, emotions and happiness. Oxygen supports cognitive function, and exercise helps to use up those excess stress hormones, so we relax, sleep and function better. Exercise is even thought to prevent dementia in old age. The worrying thing is that although we do know that exercise is good for us, we choose to live a life of physical inactivity, hoping we won't be the one to experience any consequences.

Exercise is a great way to boost energy, but so many of us don't have the energy to exercise. A survey by the Chartered Institute of Physiotherapy found that out of the 63 per cent of Britons who admitted to not doing enough exercise, 25 per cent put it down to their lack of energy. Mitochondria require oxygen to create energy and, as it's exercise that improves oxygen levels, it makes sense that the more active you are, the more energy you will have.

The problem, though, is how do you get started again, if you are inactive? Exercise is about using the body; physical activity doesn't have to mean playing competitive sport or going to the gym five times a week. It's about getting out of your chair, moving and raising your heart rate. We can incorporate exercise into our everyday lives by being active – walking upstairs, cycling to work, doing lunges as you do the hoovering – there are numerous ways to raise the heart rate and get more blood pumping.

Here are seven ideas on how to use movement to improve your energy.

1.   Practise deep breathing

Breathing, the very process of expanding your lungs with an intake of air and relaxing them again as the air is expelled, is the most natural movement we do. It plays a key role in energy production, yet we give little thought to just how powerful we could make this move.

The quality of each breath and the amount of oxygen taken in will depend on the degree to which the lungs move. Our lungs are big beasts, filling the chest cavity down to the abdomen, yet unless you're active, you have a tendency to merely breathe into the upper section of the lungs: what we call *shallow chest breathing*.

Shallow breathing is common in people who sit a lot during the day. There is little movement of the lower ribs, diaphragm and abdomen, and because of this you will not be achieving the full complement of oxygen possible. If you want to improve your energy, you need to take the time during the day to bring a deeper movement to your breath. This movement expands the intercostal muscles between the ribs, and engages the diaphragm muscle so the abdomen lowers and is pressed outwards, which provides room for the lungs to expand to full capacity, using both the upper and lower portions of the lungs.

This lung workout should be practised three times a day: morning, at noon and in the evening. Practising this will improve your lung movement capability, your oxygen efficiency and your energy, so with every breath you take you inhale more oxygen.

Simply sit comfortably on a chair with your feet on the floor in front of you and your hands on your lap or belly, and take ten conscious deep breaths, where you draw air deeply into your lungs from top to bottom so your belly rises, then empty your lungs from bottom to top. Breathe in slowly for the count of four, hold your breath for four, then breathe out for the count of eight. As you finish your out-breath, draw your abdomen back towards your spine.

If you prefer to stand up, you could bring even more movement into this exercise by raising your arms on each in-breath and lowering them on an out-breath.

2.   Don't just sit there, do something!

I could use this chapter to promote the virtues of sport, team games, running marathons and so on; but, to be honest, if you are someone who already does this and knows only too well the positive effects being so active is having on your physical and mental health and, of course, your energy, then I'm merely preaching to the converted.

If, on the other hand, you don't move much, yet you're desperate for more energy, you need to find ways to incorporate movement into your life. I appreciate it may not be quite so straightforward as that. Any form of exercise is associated with being fit, body-confident and nimble on your feet, which may not be as you see yourself.

You have to begin somewhere. Sitting for long stretches of time slows your metabolism, blood circulatory system and brain function. Not only will you not be performing at your best, but it's also a health hazard. You cannot hope to feel alive and brimming with vitality if all you do is sit.

Here is my advice. Set an alarm on your phone, and every fifty-five minutes stand up and walk about for five minutes. Swing your arms up and down. Kick your legs forward and then backwards to kick your backside, then swing your arms from side to side to free up your abdomen. Do this every hour of your waking day when you are inactive. This means during the day at work, and during the evening at home when you are slumped in a chair watching television or on your phone.

That is way better than doing nothing! It will boost your circulation and re-energise you.

3.   Get up and walk more!

Expert opinion tells us now that walking is a valuable way to increase energy. It is easy and straightforward. You can do it at your own pace, in a place of your choice, even your own garden if you don't want to be out in public; you don't need any specialist equipment, and it's *free*! What's not to like?

A twenty-minute brisk walk lowers elevated stress hormones, lifts your mood, improves your focus and concentration, and increases energy for the next two hours. This means a walk in the morning on the way to work, one at lunchtime and another in the evening has the potential to keep you energised throughout the day, and that doesn't even take into account the physical benefits it provides.

If you are new to walking, start with a leisurely fifteen-minute walk every day, and over six weeks build up to a thirty-minute walk. As you build up the time and speed, be conscious of your posture. Stand tall, with your shoulders relaxed and in line with your hips. Engage your core muscles by holding your tummy muscles in, tightening your buttocks and tilting your pelvis slightly forward. Bend your arms to slightly less than 90 degrees, and swing them rhythmically back and forth as you walk. As you increase your pace, take smaller steps to maintain your balance.

Devise a plan for you to follow that keeps you motivated and eventually takes you to walking for thirty minutes, five days a week. Plan for a five-minute warm-up and five-minute cool-down. Start with a few minutes of slowish walking, followed by brisker walking that raises your heart rate. Each time you increase the length of time you walk for, increase it by five minutes and maintain this for one week.

Week	Warm-up	Brisk walking	Cool-down	Total time
Week 1	5 minutes	5 minutes	5 minutes	15 minutes
Week 2	5 minutes	8 minutes	5 minutes	18 minutes
Week 3	5 minutes	11 minutes	5 minutes	21 minutes
Week 4	5 minutes	14 minutes	5 minutes	24 minutes
Week 5	5 minutes	17 minutes	5 minutes	27 minutes
Week 6	5 minutes	20 minutes	5 minutes	30 minutes

If you really want to switch off, listen to some music or a podcast, or even learn a language while you walk. The mind is a wonderful thing, and the chances are it will be subconsciously solving a problem for you while you're engaged in walking. The extra daylight will also help you sleep better later.

High-intensity interval training is all the rage as a way to improve fitness. Once you have built up to thirty minutes and feel comfortable and confident doing this, you can add some quick bursts of speed or hill walking into your walking plan. Start with your regular warm-up walk. Then bring in cycles of sixty seconds of brisk walking, using your arms to pump you along, followed by three to five minutes of gentler walking into your brisk walking activity. Finish with a cool-down and stretch of your calves, hamstrings, arms and neck.

If you want to take your walking to a new level, try Nordic walking, where you walk with poles. It looks rather like cross-country skiing, and that's because it was developed in Finland to enable cross-country skiers to train throughout the year! Holding poles means your arms swing more and your stride is longer, providing the body with an even greater workout.

The Ramblers Association website will tell you about walks they organise in your area. And if you really get the walking bug (as I have), possibly set yourself a goal to walk one of our nineteen national trails (*www.nationaltrail.co.uk*) and sign up for a charity fundraising walking event such as the MoonWalk, which involves walking the

River Thames bridges in London, or even an international challenge such as walking the Great Wall of China or Machu Picchu in Peru.

Rob's story

Rob had a demanding job as a marketing director. He had a team of eight people reporting to him, and he reported directly into the Chief Executive. Rob typically worked ten-hour days and had a long commute on top of this. He left home very early in the morning, and arrived back exhausted and filled with guilt that yet another week had gone by when he hadn't seen much of his young children.

For months the children had pestered for a dog, and when this little ball of fluff arrived it really irritated him – he didn't have time for this.

Rob came to see me, as he felt he was struggling to cope. Two things struck me when I met Rob, in addition to his poor diet during the working week: he did no exercise during the week, and he felt guilty that what little he saw of his family was marred by him being tired and irritable.

Rob needed to find a way to bring more movement into his life, but not in a way that kept him away from the family home for any longer than he already experienced. We looked at changes that could be made to Rob's diet, and I also made one lifestyle change. When he got home from work each evening, he was to change out of his work clothes and take the dog for a thirty-minute walk.

Despite Rob's shock at such a suggestion, he tried it, and he was amazed at what it did for him. He was so focused on not losing this young dog, he had little time to think about work and the day's issues. He would come back home more refreshed and energised. His sense of humour returned, and more importantly he felt able to engage with his family. He was more energised and effective.

Part 2

4. Bring movement into your work life

The workplace is a sedentary box. Hours are spent in a state of inactivity, and excuses are prolific when it comes to being active. The most frequent one I hear about is being too busy to go to the gym. Let me tell you, there is no excuse! There are plenty of opportunities to bring movement into you working life. And if you do want to go to the gym, or go for a swim, all you have to do is schedule it into your diary and not allow anything to supersede it. You'll be more productive for having that time out.

Your day starts with your commute. What can you do to travel under your own steam? Could you cycle some of the way? How about parking your car in a car park further away from your office than your usual one? How about leaving your car at home periodically and getting public transport to work? If you do take public transport, get off a stop or two earlier and walk in. Walking improves fitness, particularly if you walk fast enough to become slightly breathless. It also improves cognitive ability and helps to reduce excess stress hormones, which in turn help your creativity. You will be much more productive.

When you arrive at the office, shun the lift and head for the stairs. Walking up is good, but you can boost your fitness by building up to running some or all of the flights. If you push off with your foot flat on the floor rather than on tiptoes, you will use your body weight to work your muscles more.

Once at your desk, set an alarm to get you moving for five minutes in every hour. This is your 'energy time'. Energy time is particularly important when you're working on a very intense piece of work that requires focus. Stand up and do some calf raises, squats or knee lifts, or lock your hands behind your back and stretch your shoulders out. You could walk around the office for five minutes, or even go to the stairs and run up and down a couple of flights.

Use the energy time to do some desk exercises. You could stretch your hands out in front of you; or lean against the backrest with your hands behind your neck, stretching out your elbows; or use the armrest to twist your body to one side then the other. Do knee lifts from a seated position, or do leg raises with your legs straight out in front of you, or circle your ankles.

There's no need to bring water with you to work. Use your energy time to go to the water cooler and top up your bottle, or be the one who offers to go out to get some hot drinks.

When lunchtime comes, get outside and take a walk.

Be active when you're standing, maybe when you are waiting for the printer to finish some printing or the kettle to boil. Try balancing on one leg, then the other. All you have to do is lift one foot a little off the ground, then move to the other foot. Balancing postures require you to engage muscles all over the body, which increases the blood supply to them and boosts energy.

If your energy drops during the day, find a quiet spot to do some deep diaphragm breathing – just three deep breaths can energise you.

There is absolutely no excuse for not increasing the amount you move during your working day.

5. Power up your home routine

I'm sure there is plenty to do when you're home from work, and you most likely have a to-do list for the next bank holiday weekend, including projects that may involve decorating or gardening. If you're low on energy, your heart may sink at the very thought of it. That's no excuse for not bringing some movement into some of the more routine things you do at home.

Here are a few ideas – you never know, they may even make it more fun: a double boost for your energy!

• While waiting for the kettle or a pan of water to boil, do some press-ups using the kitchen worktop to support you. Add in a few squats or star jumps.

- While dinner is cooking, put a baked bean tin in each hand and do some arm exercises, or use a sport elastic band or dumb-bell if you have one. Resistance is good for strength and tone.
- Do some squats while brushing your teeth.
- Use the time doing housework to add in some exercises – lunges while using the vacuum cleaner or sweeping, heel raises while dusting, side stretches while cleaning windows.
- Do some exercise by following a YouTube video rather than sitting watching mindless television.
- At the supermarket, park as far away as possible and carry your shopping back to the car.
- When you get up in the morning, give yourself time to do some stretching exercises or arm circles to loosen up the neck and shoulders.
- Instead of leaving things that need putting away upstairs at the bottom of the stairs until there is enough to make a trip worthwhile, just go for it with each item. Run up the stairs, gradually increasing your pace from walking gently to running as fast as you can. If you have a bit of free time, do this for five minutes, building up to ten minutes.

6. Find an activity that boosts your oxygen intake

There's a wealth of research coming though that tells us that any type of movement that raises your heart rate and gets you sweating for a sustained period of time has a significant impact on your brain. Fire up your brain and fire up your energy.

Movement doesn't just mean the gym. It's also not just about the activities we hear so much about: jogging, cycling or swimming.

If the thought of these fills you with horror right now, there are other options. It's about finding an activity that works for you, and there's quite an assortment to choose from. Check out classes at your local sports centre, village hall or adult education centre. These may include yoga, Pilates, dance classes such as Zumba, FitSteps, ballet and ballroom. There are walking groups (check out the Ramblers Association). How about an exercise bike? It's a great way to practise high-intensity interval training. Put it in the living room and go on it while watching your favourite television programme or the news.

You should be doing 150 minutes of activity each week, spread over three sessions – but if this is not possible for you, anything is better than nothing. Try for two sessions spread out by a few days, so you have time to recover; and if it helps, mix and match sessions so you don't get bored.

When you start, don't go so crazy you injure yourself or give up easily. Just go at a moderate pace to begin with, building up to a point where you can still just talk when you carry out your activity. Keep a diary to track your progress so you can see how far you have come. Or invest in an activity tracker, if you prefer a gadget to a diary.

Have a workout buddy to go with you. That way, you keep each other motivated. You could even share a personal trainer with a friend or colleague to reduce the costs.

Part 2

7.   Use technology to track your movement

There's a whole plethora of technology out there that watches out for your movement, including free 'apps' for your phone.

A simple pedometer is a great way to motivate you to get moving. The recommendation is 10,000 steps over the course of the day until you go to bed, but you may need to start lower than this: 2000 or 5000. Set yourself a target each week, gradually increasing the number of steps you do, and look for every opportunity you can find to walk.

Using the stairs rather than the lift is one. Going to speak to someone rather than emailing is another.

If you want something more sophisticated, try a fitness tracker (or fitness band). They vary in functionality from a simple step counter to a device that does it all, including tracking heart rate for elite athletes. They are not 100 per cent accurate, but they give you a guide and they are a lot of fun.

Activities to learn more about how far movement optimises your energy

Activity 1: The power of breath

Try the following breathing exercise.

1. Sit comfortably on a chair – not a bed or you will fall asleep (unless you want to do this).
2. Think about how you feel sitting on the chair. Where are your feet placed, and how do they feel? What about your buttocks on the seat of the chair? How does your back feel against the chair? How are your shoulders feeling, and your head and neck on your shoulders?
3. Now concentrate on your breathing. Where are you breathing? In the shallow upper part of your chest or deep into your belly?
4. Place your hand on your belly, relax your jaw, then take a deep breath in through your nose for the count of four. You should notice your belly rise up. If it's difficult to breathe through your nose, breathe through your mouth.
5. As soon as the breath finishes, breathe out for the count of eight and notice your hands fall. As you reach the end of the breath, pull your stomach back towards your spine. This will allow you to exhale the last bit of air.

6. Continue with deep belly breaths, focusing your mind on the inhale and exhale in rhythmic movement, with the out-breath lasting twice as long as the in-breath. If you find it difficult to think of your breath, think about a wave coming into the shore then going out again.
7. Do this for about two minutes. Then return to gentle breathing.
8. Repeat this exercise every evening when you arrive home from work.

Activity 2: What activities have you done in the last week to raise your heart rate?
Consider all activity, such as playing football, going to the gym, swimming, dancing and tennis, as well as taking the stairs instead of the lift, walking to the shops and doing morning stretches.

Part 2

Day	During the day	In the evening
Monday		
Tuesday		
Wednesday		
Thursday		
Friday		
Saturday		
Sunday		

Activity 3: What could you do to become more active?

Our level of physical activity is only a third of what it was fifty years ago. Although our jobs are not as physical as they were, it's important that you don't just spend your day sitting: sitting at a desk all day, sitting on public transport or in your car as you commute, and sitting on the sofa in the evening.

1. Identify how you can incorporate exercise into your daily life.
2. What rituals will you put in place to make sure you stick to your plans?

What I could do to exercise more	How I will ensure I stick to it

Part 2

Activity 4: Your walking plan

As described earlier in this chapter, devise a plan for your walking programme. Make sure you take into account your current level of fitness and any injuries. How will you reward yourself when you have reached your target?

Week	Warm-up	Brisk walking	Cool-down	Total time
Week 1				
Week 2				
Week 3				
Week 4				
Week 5				
Week 6				

Activity 5: Your activity planner

Record your activity plan. Record the activity you will do (walking, jogging, marching, swimming, cross-trainer, strength training, resistance training, lunges, jumping jacks), the pace (slow, medium, fast), duration, and rest days.

Part

2

Week	Mon	Tue	Wed	Thu	Fri	Sat	Sun
1							
2							
3							
4							
5							
6							

Your reflections

What has resonated with you while reading Step 3: Movement for optimum energy?

- What have you learned about yourself?
- What have you learned about the state of your energy?
- What have you learned about the reasons for your low energy?
- What do you need to start doing that you have not done before?
- What other thoughts do you have?

CHAPTER 7

Step 4: Connectivity for optimum energy

◊ Do you believe that you get more done by being on your own?
◊ Do you prefer not to talk to or engage with colleagues in case they expect something from you?
◊ Do you focus so much on your work that you spend little time socialising?
◊ Do you find you have no time for interests and hobbies outside of work?
◊ Do you find people an unnecessary distraction?
◊ Do you lack the energy to listen to someone else's problems right now?
◊ Are you insensitive to other people's emotions?

If you answered "Yes" to any of these questions, you should pay special attention to this section.

People need people! We are social animals who rely on connecting with others for our survival. But human contact isn't just about surviving, it's also about thriving. The giving and receiving of attention feeds our reward system and makes us feel stronger and happier. When we are connected we're healthier, we experience fewer depressive symptoms and we live longer, healthier lives.

Socialising is an incredibly powerful way to boost your energy. Scientists suggest that it's all down to the stimulation of activity in the brain, which keeps us focused, alert and responsive and stimulates our nervous system. It's exercise for our minds! It fires up the release of chemical messengers such as dopamine and serotonin, which are known for improving mood and boosting energy, but it also has one more very powerful effect.

Socialising triggers the release of a neuropeptide, *oxytocin*. This is the love and bonding neurochemical which makes us feel more attached and gives us that 'feel-good' feeling. As you are all too aware, a good time spent socialising can mean that 'feel-good' feeling lasts for quite some time.

Have you ever had a great night out with friends and still felt in high spirits the next day, despite what pressures you're experiencing? Well, that's because oxytocin also raises serotonin levels. It's thought that serotonin-producing neurones also have oxytocin receptors, so when oxytocin is released, it attaches to the receptors on the serotonin neurones, triggering the release of serotonin.

Socialising is more important than ever. Many of us no longer live in close proximity to our families, or work from home and are isolated from our colleagues, or commute long distances to work. We have to make even more effort now to socialise. Prolonged social isolation, with no beneficial gain, is physically, mentally and emotionally harmful. It triggers negative thoughts, emotions and feelings, so the more you isolate yourself, the more anxious, depressed and low you will feel.

1.   Mix with high-energy, positive people

When the time you have available to socialise is in short supply, if you want to get every chance you can to restore your energy, you should surround yourself with the people who mean something to you. This means people who are positive and upbeat, who make you feel good, both in the situation and about yourself.

Avoid like the plague the ones you find irritating or painful, who suck your energy from you. The doubting, negative complainers who criticise and gossip. The ones who are constantly competing for attention or to be top dog, and who rock your self-esteem.

As soon as you feel your mood slipping or energy dropping, seek out the high-energy people. Head for the water cooler or kitchen, or maybe nip downstairs to chat with the people at reception. If this isn't possible, take yourself off to a lively café and people-watch.

Be extra careful if you're a lone home worker. You can get used to the isolation, and it isn't good for your mind. Too much time alone reduces creative thinking. Creativity boosts energy, so find someone to go for a walk with at lunchtime, or make sure you call someone during the day who you'll be able to have a lively chat with.

If you're an introvert, this may all sound a bit too extroverted for you. You may be feeling that the last thing you need is social contact with people, particularly high-energy, gregarious extroverts. Think again. It's not that you don't need it, it's just that you prefer a certain type of social contact. One where you can talk in depth about a subject, rather than having to engage in small talk. You still need contact – you just have to seek out the type that suits you best. And, if it does mean a lively event filled with chatter, prepare a few things you could start a conversation with. If all else fails, stand and smile. The very nature of smiling can give your energy a boost.

Part 2

2. Find more opportunities to socialise

The opportunities to socialise may not always be obvious, and with everyone so busy right now, you cannot always rely on others to instigate something.

Ali's story

Ali worked as a copywriter for an organisation which was going through a lot of change. The company had recently been taken over by another company, and it was a worry, as he liked his work life to be straightforward and stable. The new parent company had a very different culture, and he was concerned that they would look at him and decide that he didn't fit and make him redundant. He was in the process of buying a flat and couldn't afford for this to happen.

Ali decided that the best thing he could do was to hide away and just do his job without drawing any attention to himself. This worked well until his department moved into new premises in the parent company, where everyone was expected to hot-desk. He soon found out that hot-desking wasn't too much of an issue, as people tended to make claim to a certain desk, and it was really only the people who worked remotely most of the time that had a problem.

Ali found a quiet spot, away from his colleagues, and continued to keep his head down. He had noticed that he didn't seem to be as creative as he usually was, but was pretty sure that this was only because his mind was distracted by the changes and his concerns for his future.

What Ali hadn't bargained for was that it was this drop in performance that flagged him up to his manager. At his next review, his manager highlighted his disappointment in his performance over the last few months and mentioned that he'd noticed Ali wasn't mixing as much with his colleagues.

Luckily for Ali, his manager was insightful and suggested that it was his lack of connection with people that was stifling his creativity. If he wanted to improve his performance, he had to interact with others more. By feeding off their positive energy, he would grow his energy and his creativity would return. This made sense to Ali, and it was only as he connected more that he realised just how badly distancing himself had affected his energy and his performance.

Five years ago, I was becoming fairly frustrated that I had little opportunity to socialise. In addition to being a wife and mum, I was also travelling a lot with work and I had become a trustee of a large charity. Yes, I was busy, but what was more of a problem was that I was just too exhausted to take the lead. I loved walking the dog, and the previous year had joined a friend as she embarked on a walking project. The idea of walking a national trail appealed to me. I emailed some of my close friends to ask whether anyone was interested in joining me. It was one of the best decisions in my life. It was the start of a walking group that has seen us walk six national trails and explore so much of my local area. We have exercised our legs and minds. Laughed so much. Supported each other when experiencing difficulties, and, more than anything, it brought a sense of balance back into my life.

Think about what you can do to become more social with your partner, your family or your friends, or even individually. Could you set up a book club, sports team, theatre club or knit-and-natter group? If you don't want too much social connection, what about taking up a new hobby or becoming a volunteer for a charity? Volunteering boosts serotonin and dopamine, something work might not be doing right now! Even walking a neighbour's dog or taking the kids to the park with a ball or skipping rope brings you into contact with people.

Give it some thought. It changed my life in more ways than I ever expected.

Part
2

3.   Schedule social events in your diary

A busy life filled with too many demands and pressures can make it difficult for you to keep in touch with friends and family. To a certain degree, social media has made it easier to touch base, but you can spend a lot of time making promises to get together and never actually schedule anything.

You need to make your diary a 'life' diary. It should not be limited to work appointments but should include every part of your life. I schedule into mine the time I speak to friends; events I might need to plan for, such as getting the girls together to celebrate someone's birthday; when I'll walk the dog; and when I can have someone over for a cuppa. Every public event I see mentioned in my local paper I pencil in, and closer to the time I review whether I want to go to it and who could join us. Once you've added in all of the sports and recreational activities you do, your diary can look pretty full – *but* the upside is that it isn't all about work.

4. Develop your empathy skills

Generating strong relationships is far from easy. People are complex and idiosyncratic. Each of us has our own expectations and ways of doing things, which can change with the wind. You can't always expect people to treat you in the way you would like to be treated, so you need to take control of the relationship yourself. By communicating well, listening attentively, showing empathy, you will soon become adept at interacting with others.

Good relationships start with empathy. Empathy is where you get on the right wavelength with someone. You put yourself in their shoes and identify with and understand the other person's situation, feelings and motives.

Empathy begins with attentively tuning in to the person you are interacting with and using the information you glean from them, to act with consideration towards them. It requires active listening, whereby you not only listen to their words, but you show genuine interest in understanding what the other person thinks, feels or wants.

Empathy is a powerful route to creating positive relationships and connection. There's a quote by the poet and activist Maya Angelou which captures it perfectly: "People will forget what you said, people will forget what you did, but people will never forget how you made them feel."

5.   Deal with difficult people

Difficult people can soon get on your nerves, and if you let your feelings fester they'll rob your energy as well. If you can't avoid these people, you need to deal with how they make you feel. Take comfort that other people may also know they are difficult – it's not just you. On the other hand, *they* may find *you* a difficult person. People respond in kind, so whatever your course of action, you must ask yourself about the part you play.

Stay calm, bide your time and, when you are ready, take action. It helps to prepare for this. Start by thinking why they are difficult. If it's your manager, is it because he takes your ideas, or he wants everything done his way, or maybe she micromanages you? If it's an acquaintance (I stall at saying 'friend'), is it because you feel you don't have an opinion or they publicly put you down?

Your best starting point is to probe. They have made a statement: ask them to explain why. "That's interesting – why do you think that?" In many cases, if you probe enough, it makes them back off.

The worst thing you can do is to get emotional or angry and tell them outright why they are so awful. It helps to prepare for difficult conversations in advance and practise what you want to say in the mirror to build your confidence. When you meet the other party, acknowledge their point of view first before you share yours, then look to how you can solve the situation and move on.

Be aware that you cannot change people, only yourself, so be brave and be part of the solution and not the problem; others will notice and respect you for this.

This is not about being too 'nice' or always being the one to capitulate – certain people will exploit this. It's about being assertive

Part
2

so you still get your point across, but also about being solution-focused to reach agreement between all sides.

If you need to plan and rehearse for it, here is what you can do.

- Think about why it is you find them so difficult. What are they doing and how does it make you feel? Reflect on your own behaviour as well. Are you doing something that's making them behave the way they do? Maybe you are making silly mistakes in your work.
- Consider what you hope to accomplish by taking this up with them. Is it best brought out in the open or would it be better to let it lie?
- Prepare a conversation, where you can safely share your feelings. See Activity 4 in this chapter. Explain your issue and how it makes you feel. Use specific examples and explain why this is a problem for you. Indicate that you wish to resolve the situation and would welcome their views.
- Listen to their response to understand why the situation is as it is. Then question their response (you need to remain in control of this conversation).
- Come to an agreement on how you can move forward.

Conflict is another situation which can drain your energy. Conflict takes place when opinions, perspectives and expectations contradict each other, resulting in disagreement or dispute. If you are going to build positive connections, you need to manage conflict. This means that you need to prevent conflict occurring in the first place, and that starts with how you perceive the situation. When conflict occurs, try not to take what someone has said personally. Instead, use your empathy skills to understand their perspective. So often, angry people calm down when they believe that they are being listened to. And when all else fails, it may be that you have to say, "Let's agree to disagree agreeably."

6.   Get out and network

Networking is a way to broaden your contacts. Relationships are not just for social reasons. You can gain a lot from a working, transactional relationship with a person who you are less likely to socialise with. There are two variants of transactional relationships: internal and external contacts.

Internal contacts come from within the organisation you work for. They are the people you could draw on any time you need information, resources or access to other people. You develop these by socialising at work, attending internal events such as presentations and workshops, and using them to get to know the person sitting next to you, someone you don't know. You also develop them by offering to do something for someone in return for what you would like them to assist you with. We call this *reciprocity*.

External contacts are gathered from actively going out and meeting people, whether by attending or speaking at a conference, or a networking event held by your professional association or trade body. You can join round-table forums as a representative of your company, offer your company as host for an event or write to someone you admire in your industry (flattery always works). Employers love to hire people with connections, so developing an internal and an external network is a valuable asset in your career.

The trick is to collect contact details whenever you meet someone new. Do not be shy or embarrassed asking for this – all successful business people do it. Do not limit your network just to people you are 'friends' with or already have a business relationship with. Look beyond these people to anyone you have made even the briefest acquaintance with, at a meeting – it might be a customer, a professional contact or an industry specialist. The important thing is to think of it like throwing out a net to the people who work in your industry.

Part
2

7.   Give people your attention

Being attentive means paying close attention to someone. It is the most powerful attribute in making a connection with another person.

You begin by giving them your absolute attention. Show them that you are interested in them by asking a powerful question that is relevant to them. If they looked tanned, ask if they have been on holiday. If you haven't seen them for a while, ask them if they've had some time off.

If all you ask is how they are, they're likely to reply "fine"; so when they ask you (if they do), you'll say "fine", and that brings the whole sorry interaction to a close. What have you gained? I would suggest nothing, because FINE merely means 'Feelings Inside Not Expressed'. By asking a powerful question, you begin to gain an insight into who they are and what their interests are.

You then actively listen. Active listening means listening behind the words and between the words to what is actually being said and what it means. It requires you to refrain from talking or interrupting. Most people think they are listening, but, in all truth, they are not. They are either thinking about how to make a quick getaway or pondering their next question or response.

Active listening requires you to listen, process what has been said and then respond. There is a wonderful definition by Ambrose Bierce: "Bore, n. A person who talks when you wish him to listen." Enough said!

Use attentive body language. This involves using eye contact, possibly leaning slightly forward to show your interest and nodding your head, even smiling encouragement.

Activities to learn more about how connectivity optimises your energy

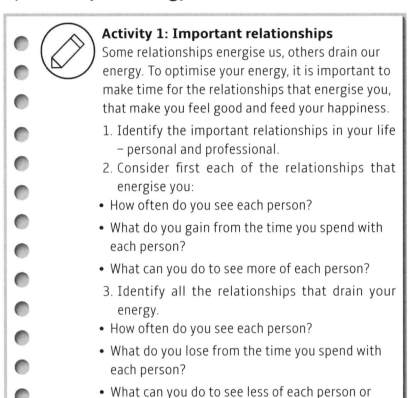

Activity 1: Important relationships

Some relationships energise us, others drain our energy. To optimise your energy, it is important to make time for the relationships that energise you, that make you feel good and feed your happiness.

1. Identify the important relationships in your life – personal and professional.
2. Consider first each of the relationships that energise you:

• How often do you see each person?

• What do you gain from the time you spend with each person?

• What can you do to see more of each person?

3. Identify all the relationships that drain your energy.

• How often do you see each person?

• What do you lose from the time you spend with each person?

• What can you do to see less of each person or manage the relationships to be more positive?

The relationships that energise me	The relationships that drain my energy

Activity 2: How empathetic are you?

1. Complete the following questionnaire about your empathy skills. Place a tick in the box that reflects the degree to which you agree with each statement, using:

   1 = Strongly disagree, 2 = Disagree, 3 = Neutral, 4 = Agree, 5 = Strongly agree

2. Add up the scores in each column, then add up these total scores to get an overall final score and record it on the chart.

Part 2

	Is this you?	1	2	3	4	5
1.	I am interested to know more about other people.					
2.	I try to understand how people think and feel.					
3.	I try to see things from the other person's point of view.					
4.	I listen and try to understand what people have to say.					
5.	I show sympathy when someone is sad or upset.					
6.	I consider the other person's feelings before saying or doing something.					
7.	I try to make people feel at ease when interacting with me.					
8.	I try to understand how and why people think and behave differently to me.					
9.	I always give my full attention to someone when they are talking to me.					
10.	I am sensitive to why something has upset someone.					
11.	Before saying or doing something, I consider how that person may feel as a result.					
12.	I allow people to tell me their point of view.					

13.	I show I appreciate the other person's view, even if I don't agree with it myself.						
14.	I remain calm and listen when someone is angry.						
15.	If there's conflict, I like to hear other people's opinions.						
16.	I can tell if someone wants to say something and I give them the opportunity to talk.						
17.	I am sensitive to how people are reacting when I am making my point.						
18.	I am aware when someone's mood is changing.						
19.	I consider the impact my decisions may have on other people.						
20.	I control my moods and feelings.						
	Total:						
	Overall total:						

A total score of:

- 80–100 indicates that you have well-developed empathy skills.
- 60–79 indicates that your empathy skills could be improved. If you want to build strong, influential relationships, look at the statements where you scored 3 or less and consider how you could begin to practise these behaviours.
- 20–59 indicates that empathy is not one of your skills. Consider signing up for an emotional intelligence course to learn more about this subject. You could also ask for some feedback from people you know and trust on how you are perceived and what needs to change. Begin by practising just one of the skills most commonly suggested: this may be listening or showing consideration.

Part 2

If you find the concept of empathy difficult, keep a diary and each day make a record of an interaction that took place. Consider the following:

- What was the situation?
- How did I behave?
- What questions did I ask?
- What does that person think, feel, want?
- How did the interaction end?

Activity 3: Dealing with a bad boss or client

It is really miserable, and zaps your energy interacting with negative, unhelpful, toxic people.

1. Look at the list below. What behaviours do you recognise in that person (this could be your direct line manager, or someone more senior you may be working with or regularly come into contact with, or your client)?

- Focuses on themselves – it's all about them
- A win/lose mentality – has to be seen to be a winner at all costs
- Plays games with people – criticises employees in front of others
- Abuses their position – behaves well when dealing with powerful people, and badly when dealing with less powerful people
- Micromanages – won't delegate projects, authority and responsibility to help people develop
- Has a temper – gets angry and abusive with people
- Always knows best – pretends to listen and then ignores suggestions, belittles other people's ideas or just gives orders

- Fails to follow through on commitments – will agree a course of action, but then won't deliver on their actions
- Lies – will happily tell untruths if it helps them get their way or avoid responsibility
- Comes first – insists that everything has to stop to deal with their priorities
- Finds fault – blames other people for failures
- Provides no support – won't drive change to make it easier for other people to succeed
- Selfish – no concern for the effect of their demands on other people's lives.

2. What are the good points about this person? It is important to objectively focus on the actual behaviours, not your negative perception of the person. This is because once we have a negative perception of someone, that is all we want to see, so we look for further examples to quantify our negative opinion.
3. What part are you playing in the problem? Are you not pulling your weight? Are there performance or activity reasons why your boss might justifiably have an issue with your behaviour, and therefore respond in ways that you consider toxic but they consider reasonable in the circumstances?
4. If you have the misfortune to work for a toxic boss and are clear that you are not making the situation worse, what can you do? Who can you talk to in the company: HR, a director, a colleague? What about the Employee Assistance Programme helpline if your employer subscribes to one? Can you discuss the issues directly with this toxic person, letting them know what they do, how that makes you feel and how you'd prefer them to behave?

Part 2

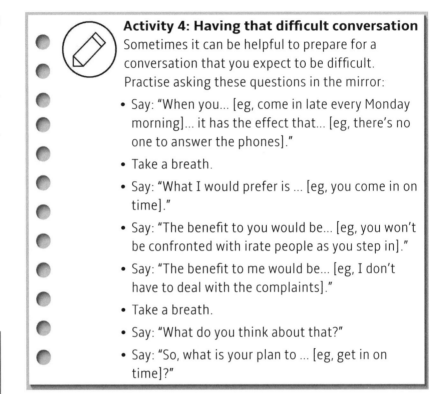

Activity 4: Having that difficult conversation
Sometimes it can be helpful to prepare for a conversation that you expect to be difficult. Practise asking these questions in the mirror:

- Say: "When you... [eg, come in late every Monday morning]... it has the effect that... [eg, there's no one to answer the phones]."
- Take a breath.
- Say: "What I would prefer is ... [eg, you come in on time]."
- Say: "The benefit to you would be... [eg, you won't be confronted with irate people as you step in]."
- Say: "The benefit to me would be... [eg, I don't have to deal with the complaints]."
- Take a breath.
- Say: "What do you think about that?"
- Say: "So, what is your plan to ... [eg, get in on time]?"

Your reflections

- What has resonated with you while reading Step 4: Connectivity for optimum energy?
- What have you learned about yourself?
- What have you learned about how connectivity impacts your energy?
- What do you need to start doing that you have not done before?
- What other thoughts do you have?

Part
2

CHAPTER 8

Step 5: Purpose for optimum energy

◊ Are you missing a purpose to your life?
◊ Have you yet to find what success and happiness really mean to you?
◊ Did you once know what you wanted from life, but do you now feel there is no point?
◊ Do the demands of work life mean that the things that are most important to you have been put on the back-burner?
◊ Do you feel as if you are no longer true to yourself?
◊ Have you lost sight of who you really are?
◊ Do you make decisions without consideration of your core values?

If you've answered "Yes" to any of these questions, pay extra special attention to this section.

Purpose is your inner self, your spirit – it's a deeper level of the energy that drives you. It's your reason for living and your strength to continue. When fully recognised and embraced, it's your motivation and passion to achieve success. Purpose is your inner flame and gives meaning to who you are.

Knowing why you do what you do and what you want to become is a crucial element of wellbeing. Having a direction in life feeds your reward system, giving you a sense of success and happiness. When you have a sense of your purpose and meaning, when you understand your purpose and live in harmony with it, you feel in tune with your inner self. As Buckminster Fuller said, "The minute you do what you really want to do, it's really a different kind of life."

We form and generate our purpose and meaning from any number of places – especially from our experiences as young children and as we grow up, and also from influential people, loved ones and the environment in which we live. We continue to develop our purpose and meaning as we tap in to the people and things that we value the most in our life, such as family, friends, professional achievement, work, and sporting success.

Analogies are frequently made about energy being the fuel in a car's tank. When we use our car, we use it to get us somewhere. Maybe we've been there before so we know how to get there. If the destination is new, we may need to use a map or our satnav. The important thing is that we have a destination we want to get to, and we need some tactics to achieve it, otherwise we'll just be driving about until we run out of fuel – and quite possibly get lost.

Part 2

The same can be said about your purpose. You need to know what it is you want: where you want to get to and how you're going to get there. This gives your life meaning and a sense of direction.

So many of us glide through life, rarely thinking about what really matters to us. How often do you think seriously and in depth about who you want to be personally, professionally, socially and even spiritually? If at one time you did know, maybe circumstances have left you feeling there's no point – it's not going to happen. But there is a point: knowing your purpose and meaning provides you with a reason for living. It boosts your self-esteem and your confidence, and gives you the resilience to deal with what life throws at you by not being distracted by life's challenges. And it's energising.

If you have never given any thought to your purpose, or maybe it's become lost or faded over time, consider the following seven steps to help you discover it or regain it, and energise your life.

1.   Know who you are

Do you know who you are? Self-awareness is such a powerful internal driver of energy, yet so many people have little idea of who they are, what their strengths, achievements and passions are, and even less of an idea of what makes them distinctive, unique and special. In other words, '*Brand You*'!

Stop for a moment and think, who is 'Brand You'? Do you know? Have you ever given any thought to it? The chances are you haven't, because we've been brainwashed into thinking that if we ever give any thought to what does make us unique and special, then we're blowing our own trumpet – and that's the surest way to alienate everyone around us. You just don't do that! But true self-awareness is not like this at all. It's not about standing on the rooftop telling everyone: it's about standing confidently and proudly and telling yourself.

Self-awareness is just that. Self-awareness means knowing who you are and acting accordingly. Self-awareness is where you can take control of your life and your emotions, and offer yourself a powerful vision of your future. It's your rudder that guides you through life. Self-awareness gives you the resilience to be able to cope with every experience that comes your way, whether good or challenging.

The funny thing is that often it's other people, particularly your nearest and dearest, who may well know a lot of the components of 'Brand You', while you struggle and are the one with a blind spot on this. I see this so frequently on workshops I run. Just identifying your personal strengths is an incredibly difficult thing to do, even for the most intelligent of people. When I explain the concept of 'Brand You', though, it really fires something up. A passion, I think: an internal flame that can become the foundation for life.

When you know what makes up 'Brand You', and regularly review it, it will influence everything you do. It's about being authentic, and that's very powerful and energising.

A good starting point is to know what your strengths are. These are your skills, talents, experiences, accomplishments and positive personality traits. Knowing them will enable you to identify your passions and motivators: what really fires you up and gets you excited. These can be powerful motivators, particularly if your self-confidence has taken a hit. Taking the leap to play to your strengths is a whole new ball game. This is where you really can grow your self-confidence, your self-esteem, your self-worth and your self-efficacy – all of which are unbelievably energising because they make you feel so fabulous.

Once you know *who* you are, it leads on nicely to understanding *why* you are (your purpose) and *what* you value the most (your core values); then *where* you want to be (your vision), *how* you will get there and *when* you will do this. These are the most important questions you can ask – it's what life is all about.

2. Identify what's important to you

As the businessman and author of *The 7 Habits of Highly Effective People*, Stephen Covey, once wrote, "Few people on their deathbed say, 'I wish I'd spent more time at work'." So why do we become locked up in a way of life that doesn't provide us with what we really want? Very often it's because we don't actually know what really matters to us – what's the most important to us. Our priorities.

You will be at your best and most energised when you are doing something that matters to you. You'll also be more focused and resilient. It will feel comfortable and natural. It will be motivating and fill you with optimism. Identifying what matters to you will provide you with a clear reason for doing what you're doing and trying to become the person you want to be – which, by its very nature, is energising. If you're doing what doesn't matter to you, I have to ask you: why is that?

Maintaining your energy in this crazy world is tough, and you need to be constantly aware of everything that has the potential to drain it. Doing what doesn't matter to you has to be way up on that list of drainers. If it doesn't matter to you, you'll be lacking all those wonderful energy-producing feelings and emotions – the feelings that motivate you and stir your passions.

To identify what matters to you, you'll need to become totally self-absorbed, and just think about yourself. What are the factors that are the most important to you? Your career? Your partner? Your health? Having an annual two-week holiday? Going for a bike ride with friends every Saturday morning? Paying off your mortgage? Passing your accountancy exams? Having a lie-in on a Sunday? The options are endless and touch every aspect of your life. Whatever they are, though, take some time to identify them. Just doing this will energise you. This 'what' question will tap in to 'who' you are and may also give you some clues as to 'why' you do what you do every day – even if it's not a pleasant thing to do. Why you get up and do a long commute. Why you endure the rudeness of your manager. Why you have to lie in on a Sunday. Once you know which things matter to you, regularly review them and consider to what extent you are allowing room for them in your life.

Aisha's story

Aisha was struggling to find any work–life balance. She worked for a leading accounting firm and was throwing everything she had into making her career a success. Initially this was exciting. She worked long hours, primarily because everyone did, and was studying for her professional exams, so learning and experiencing lots.

At college, she had set her sights on becoming a successful accountant, working her way to partner level as soon as she could. But now she'd almost lost sight of what she wanted from life – it was enough to just get through the day. She hadn't expected her working day to be governed by billing hours and client demands to such an extent that it left her with little time for anything else in her life.

Aisha attended one of my resilience workshops and highlighted at the start her need to find some work–life balance: work was getting out of control and she was losing sight of who she was – she went as far as saying that she didn't recognise herself any more. During our follow-up coaching sessions, Aisha again highlighted her frustration about having no work–life balance and her sense that she was losing her way.

Our sessions helped Aisha to realise that a work–life balance is no longer achievable. This digital age has meant that work can encroach on every corner of your life if you let it. It was now about how you balance your life between activity and recovery, what I call life-balance.

For Aisha, work was a dominating activity which left little time for recovery. So many of her friends had stopped socialising with her as she was always cancelling on them at the last minute. Aisha had begun her career with a very strong purpose and was keen to reignite this; she felt it would give her the energy she needed, but also wanted to make sure this was not at the expense of her life overall, which, as she had experienced, would deplete her energy.

Aisha spent some time identifying what and who were important to her, both in and outside work. She then considered what she wanted from life and what would give it meaning, and how she could bring these all together in a way that would reinvigorate her passion for career success and satisfy her need for connection with friends and family. Once Aisha had identified this, she became stronger and more confident standing up for her needs – they were there at the forefront of her mind.

Part
2

3.   Live according to your values

Values are your guiding principles, which work in your mind to inform your attitudes and behaviour.

Values give you an insight into the person you really are. Your values are the rules you personally want to live by (and, frequently, they are the rules you expect others to live by as well). This is because they are the principles and standards that matter most to you, and underpin what you think, say and do. They are the internal flame that drives you, and they provide direction for many of the decisions you make.

Knowing what your values are can help you to understand why you think and behave in the way that you do. You need to be able to clearly describe your core values; but, as I've seen over and over again, it can be very tough capturing them succinctly, particularly when they are not about what you would like to be like (a 'nice-to-have'), or what you 'ought to be' (because your manager is like that or it will make you look good) – it is what is important to you, at the very core of you. If you were cut in half like a stick of rock, they would be written right through you.

Stop for a minute and give this some thought. What are the things you truly value? If this is getting you nowhere, you could ask someone who knows you well to describe your qualities, and then you could summarise those qualities with a word. Or you could think about what it is in others or your employer that you really feel uncomfortable with. Is it bending the rules, or not standing up for people, or maybe being micromanaged? If so, your values could be integrity, courage and independence. An exercise in the activity section will explore this topic further.

For example, I know that one of my core values is health. I know that was with me as a teenager and has been at the centre of my life in my career and personal life. My children often quote one of my

Part 2

expressions back at me: "empty calories". I'm not obsessed with it to the extent that it becomes the absolute centre of everything I do (I eat red meat and chips), but I know it guides me, and I can see many of the decisions I have made over my life have been informed by this value.

Operating in alignment with your core values gets your attention and energises you with strength and happiness. Operate against your core values and you will feel uncomfortable, unhappy, discontented and stressed. It will sap your energy, and has the potential to take you somewhere that takes a long time to recover from.

Think about it. Have you ever worked for a company that you felt totally in harmony with? A place where you looked forward to going to work, every single day? Yes?

It's likely that its values were in alignment with yours.

Conversely, have you had times when you dreaded going to work? When you've felt you were not doing the job you really wanted to do? Perhaps you did not like the way people were treated and felt uncomfortable with the work you were asked to do. An organisation whose work culture was leading you away from the person you really are.

Which gave you the most energy? I'm sure it's the first place! If, sadly, you are in a place where you dread going to work, then you have to change things. Complaining is of no help: find something else. Life is full of choices – you just need to know who you are and what you need, and then go and find it.

4. Have a clear vision of where you want your life to go

If you don't know where you are going, you run the danger of ending up where you don't want to be.

Having a purpose is your reason for existence, and captures who you are and what you want to become and even what you would like to be remembered for. It gives meaning to your life, which fires your passion. It drives you, focuses you, and provides a sense of reward that gives meaning to who *you* are. It builds your capacity to cope by focusing your mind on the end goal rather than the short-term annoyances and deviations that get in your way.

To stand any hope of achieving your purpose, you need to plan the journey you're going to go on to achieve it. This is your vision. It gives direction in your life. The problem is that life's fast pace can mean you lack the time to give this any attention. If that is true of you, you really are in danger of ending up somewhere you don't actually want to be.

Over and over again I hear people say they would feel restricted by having a vision. But, when they are honest with themselves, it's because they know they'll never put in the effort to achieve it. They believe that 'life' will get in the way and therefore wonder, what really is the point? What they don't realise is that a vision can be so energising that you want to do whatever you can to achieve it.

Don't be tempted to confuse a vision with a goal or a dream – it's quite distinct. Goals are fixed and measured. A dream lives comfortably away in your head: it pops up periodically to give you hope, but it isn't something that you've committed yourself to. A vision provides the direction for you to achieve your purpose. It's what you really, really want to do, and you become the master of your fate. A good vision is clear, but also flexible and adaptable so you can deal with any challenges or changes in circumstances you meet on the way, such as a health issue or unexpected redundancy.

Start by identifying your purpose. What do you want to be remembered for? What is the point of your existence? In other words, *why* do you exist? Your vision will then provide you with the *how* to get there and achieve what you want to achieve. It may then help to work backwards, from where you ultimately end up to the steps required to get you there.

Achieving your vision is more likely to be successful when you work towards it in a step-by-step fashion, rather than going all out to get there in one giant step. What you do in every moment is another step towards your ultimate goal. Do this and your brain will assist you. It maintains your motivation and drive and provides a better feedback mechanism, giving you a greater sense of achievement and reward. In fact, reward yourself when you've successfully achieved each step. It also has this uncanny way of finding opportunities for you. Have you ever decided to buy a property and suddenly found that there were so many "for sale" signs about? They haven't just appeared – they were always there – but your clever mind had filtered that 'irrelevant to life' information out until it became relevant.

Flexibility is key to a vision. Circumstances change, and so do you. To keep it real, alive and energising, you should be asking yourself regularly what you really want, what you have already put in place to achieve it, and what else do you need to do. These checkpoints will bring it alive and embed it into your psyche. Rewarding yourself along the way also helps your motivation.

Be adaptable. Your vision may well change over time. In fact, it may evolve into something quite different, but at least it is giving you direction. That said, don't give up when you face the first hurdle, and don't keep changing it just because you have a new fancy. All you're doing here is drifting. Your mind will soon suss this out and stop supporting you.

Part 2

5. Do something every day you're passionate about

Passion is an intense emotion where you have an overwhelming desire for something or about doing something. It's much more than an emotion, though. It's a strong feeling of self-confidence, self-worth and self-efficacy which fires you up, motivates you and leaves you bubbling with energy. Your body language changes, the volume, pace and tone in your speech changes, and your whole body wakes up. WOW!!!

Passions give us purpose. The thing is, there are so many challenges in life today, it can be a struggle to feel anything other than dread. You crawl out of bed feeling less than optimistic for what might lie ahead. Your train is delayed. You eventually get to work and the first thing you do is go through your emails, and you're instantly filled with panic about all you have on your plate to manage that day. You're in another meeting that's going nowhere, and by lunchtime you've lost all hope and your energy has crashed. You need to get yourself out of this state as quickly as you can, and this will happen with a dose of passion.

By incorporating something you're passionate about into your everyday life at some stage in the day, you're igniting your energy and enthusiasm. It's a short moment in a dreary day that wakes you up and makes you feel more positive and optimistic. It could be starting a new hobby or picking up one you might have dropped, achieving a new milestone at the gym, or researching a topic that fires up your interest and you could tell people about.

I recently went back to a dance class I love. Dance is a passion for me. Just doing that one class each week fills me with optimism and excitement for the week ahead. The memories of the moves regularly reignite the emotions in my head, so the activity lives on for much longer than just that hour. Optimism inspires me to be more creative, to look to the positive and definitely be more resilient about what I face from day to day. It all starts with knowing what your passions are, then giving them space in your day.

6.   Be curious

Things are not always as they appear. Curiosity is about wanting to find out more. It's about keeping an open mind and asking questions.

It's a lifetime of learning, which may serve no purpose at this point in time, but you never know when it will come in handy.

Curiosity takes the tried and tested routine, which does little to enthuse and energise, to a more flexible and interesting way of being. As Alfred Lord Tennyson said, "I am a part of all that I have met." Curiosity is a strong desire to know more, which widens your horizons and makes life so much more interesting!

I have an insatiable curiosity, which feeds my mind and stokes my energy. I love to people-watch. I love to hear what people have to say on a topic: to me, we all have a right to our opinion. I love to read and I love listening to debates. Above all I love to ask questions. My sister once looked at me in shock at a wedding we were at, about why I'd asked the question I had, and said I always cut to the chase. Maybe that's practice or maybe it's just my curiosity taking over. But if I don't ask, I won't know, and I'm always interested to know. It's what's given me the knowledge to write three books, with two of them being best-sellers.

You reading my book shows curiosity, and I thank you. What I have learned through my curiosity I am passionate to share with you. How could what you learn in your daily life benefit you? I firmly believe that curiosity is the best way to grow your career.

How curious are you? My curiosity is taking over now! If you're not particularly curious, why is that? Here are what I consider the main reasons. You may have your own. Typically, a lack of curiosity is founded on fear – it's easier to keep your mind closed. Fear of what you might learn, or fear because you were discouraged from asking questions. Children are incredibly curious and ask lots of questions; they are like sponges. Sadly, as soon as they start school they lose the capacity for curiosity – maybe it comes from the need to keep thirty children quiet and under control, but it is a shame because this skill is then lost. If you reignite this skill, you will have the edge, as business leaders tell me time and time again that they can identify people with

Part 2

high potential very early on because, more than likely, they are the ones asking lots of questions.

Questions get you noticed because asking them shows your mind is open. Questions demonstrate that you're inquisitive, interested, enthusiastic and open to new experiences. Questions provide a learning opportunity that others won't necessarily get, and questions make you more creative because they provide you with choices.

It may be that you struggle to be curious. Perhaps you can identify why from the following list of obstacles to curiosity:

- Fear of what you might learn
- Looking to the negative
- A closed mind
- Not giving the time to being curious
- Too accepting of the way things are
- Over-thinking one topic
- A lack of confidence to ask
- Sceptical about other ideas or opinions

I feel so energised just writing about this topic! My recommendation to you is to take off the blinkers and develop a curiosity for the world. It all boils down to the power of asking questions. Here's what you can do to develop your curiosity.

- Practise thinking from a different perspective.
- Think of a problem and work out how you could solve it.
- Look for connections between things.
- Stop and take stock of what is going on around you.
- Start to read more: blogs, magazines, books.
- Bounce some ideas off people and take an interest in their replies.
- Ask questions.

7.   Recognise what brings you joy

We hear and read so much about happiness at the moment, and what you could be doing in your day-to-day life to make yourself happier. I'm not convinced this is the right word or even the right approach.

Happiness is something you strive for. Either you have it or you don't, or possibly you have a bit but there's still a way to go until you feel euphorically happy. It's hard to achieve, and you have to be diligent putting things in place within your life in order to achieve it. As it's something you strive for, you can find that your mood will be low and life will feel tough if you aren't achieving it.

I'm much more of a fan of 'Joy'. Joy is so much more than happiness because it is something that sits deep within you and is not dependent on external factors. Joy is about what animates you, what gives you that warm feeling – those feelings of love and gratitude that go to the centre of your very being and give you meaning.

If you want to find joy, you need to look at what you feel inside you, your very reason for living – not what you have attained. Something can cause you great pain but still bring you great joy. I find writing books painful and difficult, yet having a platform to share my knowledge and experience gives me a great sense of joy.

Happiness is just one aspect of joy. Joy comes from a variety of feelings. From pride, from relief, from humour, love, excitement, compassion and kindness. It can come from what's inside you and from what's inside others that you pick up on. It's what makes you feel a wonder with life.

Think of two situations in the last month when you felt deep joy in your heart. If this is difficult for you, look back over some photos or videos of the time when you felt happy and alive or inspired, absorbed or rewarded by an act of kindness or love. Now think about those experiences and what they did for your energy.

Part 2

The 7 steps to optimum energy

Activities to learn more about how purpose may optimise your energy

Activity 1: Your brand

1. This is your opportunity to write your brand statement. Create a short but vibrant statement about each of the following using a sentence to describe what makes you unique and valuable.

- What do you do?
- What are you good at?
- How do you add value to your employer?
- What makes you distinctive?
- What do you want to be working on or what are your career aspirations?

If you are finding this difficult to do, you're not alone. We spend very little time self-reflecting and it takes some practice to get your mind engaged on this. Think about how people describe you when they introduce you in a meeting or to a colleague.

2. Once you are happy with your brand statement, record it somewhere where you will be able to see it often. This could be on your phone, or as wallpaper on your computer. If you want it down on paper, use special paper or card, coloured pens, highlighters – whatever you would like that makes it stand out in a special way – then put it in a place that you will see regularly – behind your wardrobe door, on the fridge, in your desk.

3. Whenever you see it, rehearse it. It needs to be on the tip of your tongue at all times.

4. Use something from it as a positive intention to start each day. This will energise you and focus your mind on career success.

Part

2

Activity 2: What are the things that matter to you?

1. Think back over the last three months and identify what truly inspired you and made you feel fulfilled.
2. What specific talents and strengths made this happen?

Activity 3: What are the most important things in your life?

1. Think about your life. Who or what is an important part of it? Make a list.
2. Identify how important each item is to you. In an ideal world, how would you like to divide your time up between them? Out of a total score of 100, assign a percentage to each item.

Part 2

Activity 4: Your core values

1. What are the values that truly guide you and underpin what you think, say and do? Take some time to read the list of values in the table on the next page. Place a tick next to the values you really believe are important to you. Do not be tempted to tick the 'I ought to be' ones or the 'nice-to-haves'.

2. If you feel that an important value is missing, add it to the end of the list. If you're struggling with this activity, ask someone close to you to give you a few phrases or words that describe you and ask them to justify why. This may get you thinking and give you some clues.

Part 2

Value	✓	Value	✓	Value	✓
Achievement		Expertise		Meaningful work	
Accountability		Fairness		Money	
Advancement		Faith		Novelty	
Adventure		Fame		Originality	
Altruism		Freedom		Patience	
Authority		Friendship		Perfection	
Autonomy		Generosity		Positivity	
Balance		Goodness		Power	
Belonging		Growth		Professionalism	
Challenge		Happiness		Recognition	
Change		Harmony		Reliability	
Commitment		Health		Reputation	
Community		Helpfulness		Respect	
Compassion		Honesty		Responsibility	
Competence		Honour		Risk	
Competition		Humility		Security	
Consideration		Humour		Selflessness	
Cooperation		Inclusivity		Spirituality	
Courage		Independence		Status	
Courtesy		Individuality		Success	
Creativity		Influence		Supportiveness	
Curiosity		Innovation		Team spirit	
Decisiveness		Integrity		Thoughtfulness	
Dependability		Justice		Trust	
Determination		Kindness		Truth	
Dignity		Knowledge		Uniqueness	
Efficiency		Leadership		Unity	
Empathy		Learning		Vision	
Empowerment		Love		Wealth	
Equality		Loyalty		Wisdom	
Ethics		Mastery		Work	

3. Review the values you have ticked; pick six values that absolutely represent who you are and record them below.
4. From the six you have selected, choose the three that are most important to you; then identify the most important, and the second and third most important. Record them in the second table below.
5. Then define what each value in your top three means to you.

	Value
1.	
2.	
3.	
4.	
5.	
6.	

Part
2

What my values mean to me	
1.	Value:
Definition:	

2.	Value:
Definition:	

3.	Value:
Definition:	

Part
2

6. Why are these values so important to you? How do you live according to these values so people would recognise them as describing you? How does 'who you are' make a difference in your life? What influence are your values having on your career?
7. For the next week, notice when you have lived according to your values.

Activity 5: My passions
1. Make a list of the things that really fire up your positive energy and make you feel alive!
2. Identify your top three in order of priority.

Passions: list below everything you are passionate about	Identify your top 3

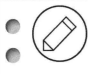

Activity 6: Who are you?

The aim of this exercise is to identify your long-term purpose.

1. Review what you have recorded in the previous exercises in this section. What is it telling you? Summarise what you have learned from these exercises.

What the previous exercises tell me

2. Imagine you are creating a chalk picture on a paving slab depicting your ideal life. What would you like your life to look like? Describe this below.

3. Imagine yourself jumping into your chalk picture, just like in the film *Mary Poppins*.

- What would the environment be like?
- What would you see?
- Who else would be there?
- How would you feel?
- What emotions would it create?
- What outcomes would it create?

Describe it in detail below.

4. Think about the following:

- How close are you to living in your chalk picture?

- Is there a significant gap from where you are now to where you would like to be?

- What do you need to do to get closer to your ideal world?

- What are the obstacles?

- How can you overcome them?

Record the answers to these in the box below.

Part 2

5. Pin your chalk picture up somewhere where you will see it every day. Regularly review it and check how far along the road you are to achieving it. If you have found it difficult to draw or describe, see if you can find a picture, saying or symbol that sums it up which you could pin up instead.

6. Don't forget to reward yourself along the way for achieving important milestones to achieving it.

Part
2

Activity 7: Your vision

1. Write down on Post-it notes every goal, dream and hope that you have. Everything that is concrete or just pie in the sky. It could be from wanting to clear out a cupboard in your bedroom to writing a novel. From chairing a meeting at work to walking the Great Wall of China. Put everything down on Post-it notes. There is no limit. You could have ten or you could have fifty.

2. Group your Post-it notes into themes covering different aspects of your life that are important to you – health, money, family, relationships, material objects, career.

3. Under each theme, sort your Post-it notes into order of preference. Tip: I use a large window or patio door to do this exercise! I can then create columns of themes.

4. Look at each theme and then review each Post-it note. Is this what you really, really want? If yes, keep the Post-it note. If no – it wouldn't bother you if you didn't do this – then bin it.

5. Make a note of what you have left, and create a timeline describing when you want to act on these goals and when you want to have achieved them by.

6. Create a plan with small steps to help you achieve your goals. Identify any limiting factors, including your own mindset and what you already have in place to drive this goal.

7. Identify who can help you and what resources you need.

8. Now off you go!

Your reflections

What has resonated with you while reading Step 5: Purpose for optimum energy?

- What have you learned about yourself?
- What have you learned about how your purpose is impacting the state of your energy?
- What do you need to start doing that you have not done before?
- What other thoughts do you have?

CHAPTER 9

Step 6: Balance for optimum energy

◊ Do you find you're juggling many different demands?

◊ Do you find your memory is not as good as it used to be?

◊ Do you find it hard to concentrate and focus?

◊ Do you worry about things more than you used to?

◊ Do you find it hard to switch off at the end of the day?

◊ Do you feel out of control with so many plates spinning?

◊ Do you feel close to burning out?

If you've answered "Yes" to any of these questions, pay extra special attention to this section. Life really doesn't have to be this way; it's very likely that you've become stuck in the 'stress' response.

Twenty-first-century living is tough. Multitasking has become an imperative, even though it's evident that it's affecting our productivity. The relentless demands on our precious time take their toll on our energy and health, and one of the first signs that you're overloaded is that you experience low energy.

We have high expectations that we can rely on our minds to just sort a way through the chaos, let us concentrate and focus, be tactical and creative, remember everything clearly and help us deliver what we need to in the best way we know possible. We feel so frustrated when this doesn't happen.

The reason we're struggling to cope is that the pressures we're experiencing continuously stimulate our stress response, resulting in high levels of the stress hormone cortisol. Cortisol does a wonderful job in focusing the mind when our 'fight or flight' response is stimulated. The problem is that the physical changes resulting from cortisol release can only be tolerated by the body for short periods of time. Today's fast-moving, multiple-demand, non-stop lives are stimulating a continuous release of cortisol, and high levels of cortisol over long periods of time are now known to be toxic for the brain, putting you in danger of being knocked off course.

Whereas we could focus and perform (to get us out of danger), now we feel irritable and anxious, and struggle making decisions. All those things we want the brain to do for us just won't happen. Worst of all, MRI scanning has found that long-term stress shrinks our brains, with the *hippocampus* region, responsible for logical reasoning, long-term memories and spatial navigation, being the most affected.

And, on top of all that, there never seems to be *enough me-time* to refuel. Think about it: even cars get an oil change and a regular service. No one expects a vehicle to run on empty, and I am sure you always give your car the best fuel you can afford.

To think clearly and feel energised, we need to find ways to manage the demands on our time. This requires us to become more aware of how we are using our time, and then ensure we balance it between activity and recovery to maintain and enhance our energy.

Achieving a balanced life

Time doesn't change, yet the amount we're expected to successfully complete in that time continues to grow. To protect us and help us deal with these demands and other pressures and worries we experience, our body uses our nervous and endocrine systems. We colloquially call this the 'fight or flight response'. It uses a part of the nervous system called the *autonomic nervous system*, and there are two parts to this: the *sympathetic nervous system* and the *parasympathetic nervous system*.

Sympathetic nervous system

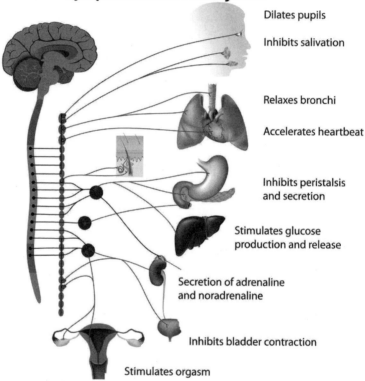

Dilates pupils

Inhibits salivation

Relaxes bronchi

Accelerates heartbeat

Inhibits peristalsis and secretion

Stimulates glucose production and release

Secretion of adrenaline and noradrenaline

Inhibits bladder contraction

Stimulates orgasm

The diagram above illustrates the sympathetic nervous system. When we experience such things as shock, fear or anxiety, it puts us on alert and physically changes the body to manage the danger. Our pupils dilate, glucose is sent to the muscles and digestion slows. After all, we don't need to grab a sandwich if we've just come face to face with a sabretooth tiger. The expectation is that this will only be for a short time.

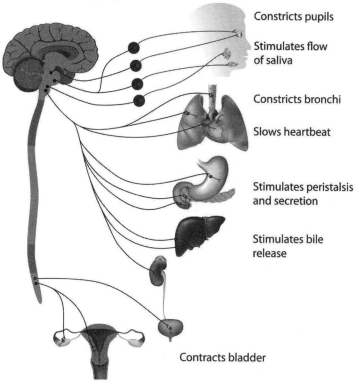

Parasympathetic nervous system

Constricts pupils

Stimulates flow of saliva

Constricts bronchi

Slows heartbeat

Stimulates peristalsis and secretion

Stimulates bile release

Contracts bladder

Part 2

As the danger passes, the parasympathetic nervous system, illustrated in the diagram above, kicks into action to return the body to its relaxed state. The heart calms and digestion begins again.

However, today's chaotic world is keeping us stuck in an 'always-doing' mode, which over-activates the sympathetic nervous system. If we get stuck here, our blood pressure is raised, and we have high levels of cholesterol and of stress hormones in the bloodstream (normal 'sympathetic' activities). We're not repairing the body, digesting our food effectively or fighting infection, which is what takes place when the parasympathetic nervous system is activated. This has a considerable effect on our energy. All 'doing' and no rest and recovery drains our batteries and puts us at risk of burning out.

Claire's story

Claire had an exceptionally busy life and rarely had a moment in her day she could call her own. She had a demanding part-time job, and she had an autistic son who attended a specialist school but lived at home. As her son approached his teens, she found coping more and more difficult.

She would wake abruptly in the night, and immediately her heart would start pounding and she would break into a hot sweat. It could take up to two hours before she got back to sleep again, if she did at all.

She was always tired and feeling tearful, and, despite having a gentle personality, was starting to get very irritable with people around her. She had been to see her doctor, who wanted to prescribe antidepressants, which Claire refused, and eventually prescribed HRT, suspecting that she was pre-menopausal even though she was in her very early forties. She willingly took it, but very soon felt worse.

By the time Claire came to see me, she was desperate. The fact that she woke in the night with a start then broke into a sweat suggested to me that she was adrenally fatigued. Claire agreed to take an Adrenal Stress Profile test, a very simple saliva test where you collect some saliva four times over your waking day.

The results showed Claire was burnt out. And, just as I had suspected, the night sweating was not a menopausal sweat, but an adrenal 'stress' sweat. I suggested some adjustments to Claire's diet and lifestyle, but my main recommendation was some adrenal support supplementation.

Six weeks later, Claire told me just what a difference this had made to her life.

Optimum energy and peak performance are reliant on resting and recovering as much as the activity itself. This means that if we're going to maintain our energy and prevent collapse, we need to put practices and rituals in place that ensure we can move successfully and appropriately between the sympathetic and parasympathetic systems.

We have grown up being trained to achieve and keep 'doing' without understanding the importance of 'undoing'. If you have been stuck in 'sympathetic' for some time, this will be difficult to achieve, not least because either you're addicted to the buzz it provides or you're too exhausted to change.

If this is the case, it will take effort, practice and tenacity – but it's imperative if you want to regain your energy. Take note, though, relaxation should not be about collapsing in a heap each evening on the sofa, but about finding ways to release tension in the body and reduce the chatter in the mind, so you create the space and energy for new activities and energy.

There's a wonderful quote from the American journalist and author Sydney J Harris: "The time to relax is when you don't have time for it." In other words, if you don't have time to switch off, you should take it as a sign that your sympathetic nervous system is becoming stuck in 'doing' mode.

Work–life balance is not really about balancing the time you spend in work with the time you spend out of work. This may come as a surprise, but, having read this far you may now understand that it's really about achieving a balance between activity and recovery. This is the balance between activating your sympathetic nervous system and activating your parasympathetic nervous system. A properly balanced life is one where we use our skills, knowledge, strengths and concentration to perform well, then allow our bodies to recharge by giving them downtime. This isn't just something confined to the end of the day when we're home from work; we need to be taking opportunities to do this throughout the day.

Part
2

1. Know how you spend your time

When you bring some sort of order to the chaos that swirls around you, you will feel more in control and less off-balance, and you will expend less energy. People think they are busier than they have ever been, but this might not actually be the case. People think they have no time for the things they really love about their life. Again, this might not be the case. To capture a picture of the true lie of the land, you need to know how you spend your time and the effect this has on your energy. Activity 1 will guide you to understand this.

Overwork is a major energy zapper. It erodes your capacity to cope and lowers your mood. I'm seeing so many people who are now addicted to 'being busy'. This is a dangerous place to be, which puts you at risk of burning out. If this is you, you need to take action. Begin by assessing your workload. Are you bored, or are you rushed off your feet with too many demands on your time? What do you actually have to do? What is within your capability to change and what isn't? Make a pact with yourself to do something about this.

2. Plan how you will use your time

If you do have more to do than time allows to get the job done, focus on what is urgent and important. Purge anything of low value. What can you free up by maybe delegating to someone else? Is it within your capacity to change the way a task is done?

Use your diary/calendar/planner to record everything you need to do in a day: meetings, priorities, deadlines, a walk around the block, trips to the gym, family commitments – this should reflect your whole life, not just your work appointments. Set up alerts to your phone as reminders and messages to stay motivated and on track.

At the end of your working day, before you leave for home, write your to-do list for the next day. Know what you want to have accomplished by the close of business the following day. This is important, because if you don't, someone else will. Prioritise your to-do list accordingly by scoring each item from one to three, where one is urgent and three is "it can wait". Make sure anything that's scored a one is a priority to complete the next day. Make sure you know your limit and what's realistically achievable, though.

Choose one priority on your to-do list and work on this as soon as you get to work in the morning, *before* you open your email ("What?!", I hear you scream). Yes, before you do anything else. Clearing this off your to-do list will trigger a huge rush of dopamine in your brain, providing a sense of achievement and reward. If you go to your emails first, you'll get sucked in and you will end up feeling out of control and fed up.

Remember: this is your day. Regularly tell yourself that *you* are in charge of your day. Tell yourself that you have choices, and take charge of those choices. This puts you in control, which is important for resilience.

3.   Take back control of digital technology

One of the biggest changes in recent years is the rise in digital technology and the way it is creating a 24/7 working culture. We are allowing these little machines to dictate to us, rather than us using them.

We spend inordinate amounts of time using digital technology in and out of work and often right up until the time we retire for bed, with activities such as reading emails or keeping up with Facebook and Twitter. If we let it, technology has the capacity to increase the length of our working day, strain our eyesight and disturb our sleep. The concentration involved certainly uses up vital energy.

Do you know how much time in a twenty-four-hour period you spend using digital technology? No? Then you really need to find out. Here are some tips on how to take back control of your digital technology.

- *Do not* look at emails, social media or anything else before you complete a priority task on your to-do list.
- Don't have your email set up to automatically inform you when an email arrives. Set aside a certain time in the day to read and respond to emails. Make sure your response is brief and you only copy in people with a direct interest in the subject matter. When an email requires a longer response, add it to your to-do list and set aside a separate time to respond. This way, you will feel you're keeping on top of your inbox and in control of technology.
- Stop checking work emails by a certain time each evening. Have an electronic sundown and put technology away two hours before bedtime.
- Have a digital-free dinner table. It will improve the interaction and conversation with your family.
- Keep a daily log of your smartphone use. There are apps to help with this, which can also limit your time on social media.
- Break your smartphone habit. Start by having a phone-free day over the weekend. Stop yourself from reaching for it when you're bored, and stop all social media notifications.

4.   Learn to say no

It's one of the biggest conundrums in the workplace. How do you say no to a request from someone when you genuinely do not have the capacity to fulfil it but you feel obliged to do so? One part of your mind is saying "Say no", the other is weighing up the consequences if you do.

These self-fabricated consequences are rarely grounded in fact. It could be that you have a belief that saying no will make the other person angry enough to put the relationship at risk. If the other party is someone more senior, you may feel obliged to agree, fearing it could put your career at risk. Or maybe it's because the feeling of guilt or being disliked is just too unpleasant to bear. The ironic thing is that absorbing these extra demands puts you at risk of burnout; and if this happens, relationships become strained, careers stall and the feelings of helplessness and despair are far worse than a momentary feeling of guilt.

It is vitally important to recognise when this 'kindness' is really about pleasing people at your own expense. You need to put yourself in control of the situation by focusing on *your* priorities – the important things you need to achieve. To enable this, you need to be aware of how the other party's request fits with your circumstances, capabilities and commitments, and then feel empowered to deal with it in a way that doesn't leave you feeling frustrated and imposed on, or worried and guilty. In other words, it's about listening and acting on your inner voice.

If something is not one of your priorities, then very politely and very straightforwardly say no. Acknowledge why you believe they have made the request, and possibly suggest an alternative, which will show you are trying to cooperate; but just keep in mind that you do not have to say yes to anything you do not have the capacity to fulfil.

Part 2

5.   Keep a stress log

Being in balance requires that you know what triggers feelings of stress. With so much going on – and if you are stressed, your judgement will be impaired – the only way to understand these triggers is to write them down.

As soon as you feel things are getting out of hand and there is more going on than you can handle, start keeping a stress log. Over a set period of time, use your log to record every challenging event and behaviour that has triggered a negative emotional response. Record the event or behaviour, what triggered it and how you responded. Look for any themes that flag up something in particular that needs addressing. If this was sorted, your life would be easier. What can you do to improve the situation?

6.   Work in sixty-minute cycles

Have you ever wondered why it is that, when you are concentrating hard on one task for a long time, one minute you are very productive and the next your mind is wandering all over the place, and you lose focus and alertness? If you try to plod on, you just don't seem to get anywhere – your energy has plummeted – but, when you take that break, you come back firing on all cylinders again. This is because our body works in a rhythmic brain-wave frequency cycle of ninety to 120 minutes, called an *ultradian rhythm*. The cycle is there to protect the brain from over-polarisation in one area of the brain. This cycle operates both day and night. During the day it determines when you will experience a state of heightened alertness, and at night it controls our REM sleep cycle, determining when we lay down memories and recharge.

This means that no matter how much we desire it, concentration does not last forever. If you take regular breaks, you will do much better in terms of energy and productivity.

The most effective way to do this is to focus on a task for fifty minutes, then take a ten-minute break when you should do something completely different. This is your recovery time, a time when you could get up from your desk and move. Take a walk up and down the stairs or outside, listen to some music or a podcast, have a chat to someone.

As you are advised to work in sixty-minute cycles, it would also help you to schedule your tasks based on these cycles and your energy levels. You may find that you are more productive and your energy is higher at certain times of the day; and tasks that require more focus, concentration and attention would be best assigned to these times. Assign more routine administrative or easier tasks to your low-energy times, when you don't feel so productive.

7.   Schedule in recovery time

If your busy life means you're stuck in 'always-on' mode, it is imperative that you take some time out to rest and recharge your energy. Without question, you should make sure you find at least fifteen minutes for yourself each day. This is your time to do something completely different and restorative.

For me, there are some incredibly powerful yoga poses that don't take too long, but never fail to boost my energy.

- If I have been sitting for a long period writing, the 'legs up the wall' posture works wonders. Sit on your bottom close to the wall, then swing your legs around and up the wall so you lie with your trunk and head on the floor. You can elevate your pelvis on a blanket, if it's comfortable. Rest your hands comfortably, then close your eyes for five to ten minutes.
- The bridge pose is a great way to energise the body and release tension. Lie on your back, arms by your side with your knees bent. Engage your core, push down through your feet and lift your tailbone off the floor, moving in one smooth movement, one vertebrae at a time. Hold the position for the count of ten. Slowly exhale and roll each vertebra back down. Repeat five times.
- The Cat-Cow posture loosens my stiff back. Kneel on all fours. Breathe in and lift your head up as you curve your back downwards. Breathe out and drop your head down as you curve your back upwards. Continue in a rhythmic breathing manner, moving gently between the cat posture and the cow posture for three to five minutes.

Part 2

If you find it hard to switch off from work when you get home, take on some rituals that create a boundary between work and home life. Ideas include:

- Stand up
- Take five deep breaths and consciously move your thoughts into home mode
- Take off your tie
- Change the glasses you wear
- On your journey home, switch from reading something connected with work to hobby reading; or stop the car on your way home and rest for five minutes, reflect on the day, then tell yourself that was then, this is now, and move consciously into home mode. For the rest of your journey, think about your family life.

Laughter really boosts energy, so make sure you have at least one fun activity on your to-do list each day.

Make sure you take your annual holiday entitlement. You need a two-week break to unwind, recharge and recover. If the demands on you are becoming too much, don't be afraid to have a discussion with your manager or HR about it. Be brave. It is better to act now than to burn out. If this concerns you, find out whether your organisation subscribes to an Employee Assistance Programme, which will have a confidential counselling helpline.

Activities to learn more about how balance optimises your energy

Activity 1: How do you spend your time?
Complete the exercises in this section as honestly as you can, and dig deep to identify what this is telling you.

1. Think about how you spend the time you have each week – this comes to 168 hours. This time is finite. You cannot bank some hours for next week or borrow for the next week. This is it.

2. Sort the activities into themes and record them on the chart below. You might like to consider time spent getting washed and dressed, eating, commuting, at work, exercise, hobbies, housework, studying and sleeping.

3. Review your chart and record your answers to the following questions in the box on the next page:

- What do you see; what is this telling you?
- How is your activity affecting your energy?
- What is the quality of your recovery time?
- What time do you take to relax and recharge your energy?
- Do these activities map with your priorities in life?

Part 2

Activity	Hours spent on this activity
	Total:

We all have time; it's how we use it that's important. This is what will either fuel your energy or drain it, and even though it may not feel like it sometimes, the balance is in your control. Give some thought to how you spend the 168 hours you have each week.

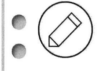

Activity 2: Energy drainers

1. What activities and events do you do each week that fuel your energy? For example, spending time with friends, reading or practising yoga.

Activities and events that fuel my energy	Activities and events that drain my energy

2. Which column is the most filled with activities and events? What does this tell you?
3. When in your week could you do more of the activities that fuel your energy?
4. What could you do to reduce the activities that drain your energy? For example, are some unnecessary? Could someone else do them?
5. Then learn to say no! If it's not one of your priorities, you don't have to say yes to anything you don't have the capacity to fulfil. Stop, take a breath, then ask yourself whether you really want to do this. If no, decline graciously and explain that you would have liked to help but you do not have the capacity right now; or, if you did do this, something else that is important for you to complete would get pushed back. Show empathy with their situation, but be firm about yours also.

Activity 3: Working with your highs and lows

1. Review Activity 1 in Chapter 2, where you looked at your energy cycle during the day. What are your high-energy times of day, and what are your low-energy times of day?

2. Think about the types of tasks you need to complete each day. When would be the best time to do them? For example:

- Times of high energy would be best utilised completing tasks that are your priority or require focus and concentration.

- Times of medium energy could be used for tasks that require moderate amounts of energy, such as hosting a team meeting or updating your manager.

- Times of low energy would be best used doing tasks such as emails, routine phone calls and travelling between offices. Tasks that do not require exceptional brain power and are more routine and repetitive than original and creative. It is not critical if you are interrupted at this time.

3. Create a framework for managing your tasks.

Time zone	How you will feel	Tasks to work on
High energy		
Medium energy		
Low energy		

Activity 4: Your digital footprint

1. How long did you spend looking at screens over the last three days? Consider your computer, tablet and mobile phone. Write your answers in the table below.

	Morning	Afternoon	Evening
Computer			
Tablet			
Mobile phone			
TV			

2. Look at your list of energy-fuelling activities in Activity 2. If you weren't spending so much time staring at a screen, what could you be doing instead that would fire up your energy? Record your ideas in the box below.

Part 2

3. What action could you take to reduce the time you spend on technology? Here are some ideas:

- Take regular breaks from your screen – five to ten minutes each hour.

- Turn off email notification and set aside a time to answer emails.

- Unsubscribe to junk email.

- Limit time on social media, and if conversations create negative thoughts, delete the application.

- Have a digital sundown, when you turn off technology a certain time before retiring for bed (preferably two hours if you do not want to disturb your sleep).

- Leave your phone and tablet in the kitchen at night, or leave them turned off. The electromagnetic waves emitted can disrupt the sleep hormone melatonin.

Activity 5: Your stress log
If life seems stressful and you're struggling to cope, it may be helpful to identify the source of your stress and the feelings and emotions that it triggers. Complete this chart for one week.

Date	Time	Stressful event or situation	How did you feel?	What did you do?	What were the consequences?

Part 2

Activity 6: Where are you in the stress response?

1. Look at the chart below and identify which column best describes you.

Part 2

	Stage 1 *Pressure*	Stage 2 *Tension and strain*	Stage 3 *Stress*
Stress	Under pressure but still feel in control	Pressure has been prolonged and I feel tense and strained	Chronic stress and close to burning out
Stress hormones	Normal on/off 'fight or flight' response	Adrenalin and cortisol levels are high	Adrenalin and cortisol levels are low despite stimulation
Response	I feel I can deal with the pressure well	I feel 'stressed', which is causing adverse mind and body symptoms, but I'm still coping	I'm now struggling to cope and respond to the pressures and demands on me
Energy	My energy is OK	I'm frequently tired	I'm experiencing chronic fatigue
Concentration	My concentration is good	My concentration is erratic	My thinking is unclear; I'm finding it hard to think straight
Memory	My memory is good	I'm struggling at times to find the right words or remember events	I feel as if my memory has shut down
Mood	My mood is good	I feel grumpy, irritable and sometimes anxious	I feel very low, detached, depressed
Sleep	OK, just sometimes the odd blip	Difficulty switching off and disturbed sleep	I'm always tired and exhausted

2. Look at the chart below and tick or underline the symptoms you are experiencing – or people have told you you're exhibiting.

Psychological and emotional signs	Physical signs	Behavioural signs
Poor concentration	Dips in energy	Workaholism
Poor memory	Tiredness and	Perfectionism
Feeling out of control	sleepiness	Making mistakes
Poor decision-making	Muscle tension	Poor time management
Worrying	Skin problems	Pushing people away
Anxiety	Indigestion/IBS	Being withdrawn
Depression	Heartburn	Relationship problems
Tearfulness	Headaches or	No time to relax
Irritability	migraines	Accident-proneness
Mood swings	Weight loss/gain	Difficulty sleeping
Low confidence	High blood pressure	Increasing alcohol
	High cholesterol	consumption /
	Heart problems	smoking
	Glucose intolerance	Change in appearance
	Diabetes	

Part 2

3. What signs and symptoms of stress do you exhibit (either you know you do or people are telling you so)?

4. How have your symptoms changed recently?

Your reflections

What has resonated with you while reading Step 6: Balance for optimum energy?

- What have you learned about yourself?
- What have you learned about how balance can affect the state of your energy?
- What do you need to start doing that you have not done before?
- What other thoughts do you have?

Part
2

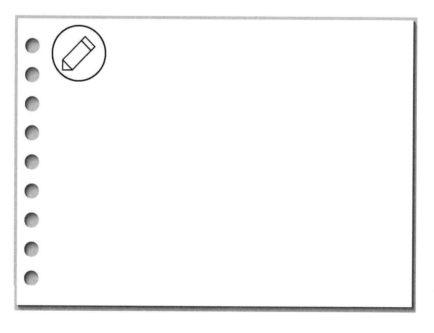

CHAPTER 10

Step 7: Positivity for optimum energy

◊ Do you have an internal critic commenting on all you do?
◊ Do you lack motivation a lot of the time?
◊ Do you find it hard to see the upside of a difficult situation?
◊ Do you have a tendency to pessimism rather than optimism?
◊ Do you feel fearful when presented with a new situation?
◊ Do you feel embarrassed to talk yourself up?
◊ Do you have a tendency to look for what could go wrong?

All too often, our mind defaults to the negative to protect us from what it perceives to be danger. The trouble is, this uses up precious energy while doing nothing to recharge you.

If you've answered "Yes" to any of these questions, pay special attention to this section.

An emotion is a strong, instinctive feeling derived from the situation you are in. It can be anything from being happy to sad, fearful to glad, cheerful to miserable, angry to serene. Positive emotions, such as delighted, proud, excited and thankful, energise and motivate you and profoundly influence the way you perform. Negative emotions draw on copious amounts of energy and drain you of your vitality.

As human beings, we have a survival mechanism that typically makes us think of the danger: the negative. If we don't control this, it can be like a warning siren which then gets stuck in the 'on' position. We default to the negative. We become demotivated, disillusioned and unhappy, all of which drain rather than replenish our energy. If you want to optimise your energy, you need to make a concerted effort to control the negative and reframe to the positive.

Within your brain you have several chemicals which are required by your brain cells (neurones) to communicate with each other and process information. These are called *neurotransmitters* and they heavily influence your emotions. They fire you up, calm you down, make you feel happy and give you a sense of reward. When they're in balance and working optimally, you have the potential to feel good and perform well. When out of balance, they can demotivate you and leave you feeling down and depressed.

The stress hormone, cortisol, has a big impact on the balance of our neurotransmitters, negatively affecting it when high. Food, blood sugar, alcohol and caffeine also affect you negatively. Neurotransmitters are mostly made from amino acids, the building blocks of protein, with some help from B vitamins to accelerate their manufacture – so what you eat is very important if you want to maintain a positive mental state.

The main neurotransmitters produced in the brain are as follows:

- **Dopamine** plays a major role in energy. It provides your drive and focus, and heavily influences your ability to experience pleasure. It's your get-up-and-go! It heightens your sense of drive, motivation, excitement and reward, and plays a key role in your ability to focus and concentrate. When dopamine is out of balance, you feel tired and apathetic, and may experience addictive disorders. Stimulants, such as caffeine, nicotine, chocolate, drugs, gambling, shopping, porn and sex, trigger the release of dopamine, giving you that perceived boost in energy and the sense of being on a

Part 2

'high'. Dopamine is made from the amino acid L-tyrosine, which is commonly found in cheese, soya, red meat, chicken, turkey, eggs, bananas, peanuts, almonds, sunflower seeds, beans, lentils and oats.

- **Serotonin** balances your mood, appetite and sleep patterns, and modulates pain. It's a nourishing chemical for the body. When levels are sufficient, you feel peaceful and happy and enjoy family, friends and your food. When they're low, you can feel depressed and anxious, worry more, struggle to sleep well and crave high-energy sweet carbohydrate foods. The body makes it by converting the amino acid L-tryptophan – which is found in abundance in chia seeds, wholegrains such as brown rice, wheat and oats, and pumpkin and sesame seeds. Fish, meat (particularly chicken and turkey), cottage cheese, yoghurt, eggs, bananas and soya also contain L-tryptophan.

- **Gamma-amino-butyric acid (GABA)** is the neurotransmitter that calms the brain down – it's your natural Valium. It's the counterbalance to dopamine and serotonin, and without it you'd be likely to experience headaches, feel agitated and have palpitations. That's because GABA relaxes and calms you and is involved in the production of endorphins, which make you feel good. It's made from glutamine, which is found in dairy products, meat, spinach, cabbage and pulses such as lentils.

- **Acetylcholine** keeps your brain sharp and alert. It helps you to process what you see, hear and feel, and to access your memories. When it's balanced, you feel alert, positive and creative. When it's low, your brain speed slows and a 'brain fog' descends: your short-term memory falters, and it becomes difficult to concentrate and follow conversations and the written word. Acetylcholine is made from choline, which is found in seafood, eggs, chicken, turkey, quinoa and almonds. Choline is one of the B vitamins, and many of us are deficient in it.

Part 2

1. Boost your brain's chemical messengers

How well your brain functions is determined, in the most part, by what you eat. I frequently hear people ask me to make them more alert and improve their memories, concentration and focus, and when I look at their food diary I instantly see that all their concerns stem from not eating the right foods – in particular, not enough protein.

If you want well-balanced neurotransmitters, you need certain amino acids from protein and a spectrum of B vitamins. If your diet is low on protein (dairy, fish, meat or eggs), wholegrains and fresh fruit and vegetables, you will not be able to make these vital chemicals.

Part 2

Dopamine	
Take note! Caffeine, sugar, nicotine and fatty foods will be very effective at increasing dopamine because they provide a sense of reward and pleasure. But this is only a temporary boost, which leaves you low on dopamine in the long run. Don't be tempted!	
Dopamine is made from L-tyrosine, found in:	
• Red meat • Chicken and turkey • Eggs • Dairy • Soybeans • Grains • Beets	• Bananas • Kiwi • Avocados • Almonds • Nuts (walnuts, almonds, peanuts) • Sunflower seeds • Beans and lentils
To convert L-tyrosine to dopamine you require: • Vitamin B6 (wholegrains, meat, dairy, leafy green vegetables, sunflower seeds, pulses) • Folic acid (wholegrains, asparagus, Brussels sprouts, cabbage, peas, spinach, pulses) • Magnesium (wholegrains, artichokes, nuts, seeds, tofu, dark green vegetables, meat) • Iron (red meat, leafy green vegetables, fish, eggs, wholegrains, beans) • Zinc (eggs, dairy, chicken, pumpkin seeds, oats, oysters)	
You can boost dopamine levels by supplementing with L-tyrosine and B vitamins. Siberian ginseng can help by supporting the stress cycle, and I particularly like the herb Rhodiola, which also supports the adrenal glands.	

- 500–1000mg L-tyrosine on an empty stomach first thing in the morning
- Take a B Complex supplement daily, providing 25mg of all the B vitamins
- 200–400mg Siberian ginseng daily with meals for two months maximum, or 200–300mg Rhodiola daily with meals

Serotonin

Take note! All amino acids compete to be absorbed into the brain. Eating some carbohydrate with L-tyrosine-rich foods will trigger insulin, which will help it into the brain. All you need is an oatcake or some bread.

Serotonin is made from L-tryptophan, found in:

• Chicken	• Banana
• Fish	• Whole grains (brown rice, wheat
• Eggs	and oats)
• Turkey	• Chia seeds
• Cottage cheese	• Pumpkin and sesame seeds
• Yoghurt	• Soybean

To convert L-tryptophan to serotonin you require:
- Vitamin B6 (wholegrains, meat, dairy, leafy green vegetables, sunflower seeds, pulses)
- Folic acid (wholegrains, asparagus, Brussels sprouts, cabbage, peas, spinach, pulses)
- Vitamin C (citrus fruit, kiwi, kale, peppers, watercress, spinach, tomatoes)
- Magnesium (wholegrains, artichokes, nuts, seeds, tofu, dark green vegetables, meat)
- Calcium (dairy, spinach, sardines, almonds, tofu, leafy green vegetables)
- Iron (red meat, leafy green vegetables, fish, eggs, wholegrains, beans)

You can boost serotonin further by supplementing with L-tryptophan, but I find 5HTP better (it is important to avoid 5HTP if you are taking any depression or anxiety prescription medication). Magnesium and folate (5-MTHF) also help support the conversion of L-tryptophan to serotonin.

- 100–300mg 5-HTP, starting with 50mg twice a day, with second dose one hour before bed, building up gradually
- Vitamin B Complex supplement daily, providing 25mg of all the B vitamins, or 400–800mcg Folic acid with meals daily
- 400mg calcium and 400mg magnesium with meals daily

GABA

Take note! A good gut microbiome is important, as bacteria help to convert glutamine into GABA. Stimulating the conversion of GABA requires you to switch off the 'always-on' lifestyle and train yourself to relax.

Part
2

The following can help:
- Eat fermented food such as live yoghurt, kefir and sauerkraut
- Mindfulness meditation
- Deep-breathing exercises
- Walking, yoga or gentle exercise
- Epsom salt baths (which contain magnesium)

GABA is made from glutamine, found in:

• Meat • Dairy • Potatoes • Spinach	• Cabbage • Beans and lentils • Wheat

To convert glutamine to GABA, you require:
- Vitamin B6 (wholegrains, meat, dairy, leafy green vegetables, sunflower seeds, pulses)
- Magnesium (wholegrains, artichokes, nuts, seeds, tofu, dark green vegetables, meat)

Supplementing with GABA is illegal in the UK. L-theanine (found in tea), taurine and magnesium are helpful in relaxing and calming the mind and body – or calming herbs such as valerian, hops and passionflower.
- 1000mg L-glutamine daily, and gradually increase to a maximum of 5000mg providing it does not cause diarrhoea
- 300–600mg taurine twice daily, away from food
- Vitamin B Complex supplement daily, providing 25mg of all the B vitamins
- 300mg magnesium twice a day with food
- 50–100mg valerian two to three times a day (third dose just before bed), away from food

Acetylcholine

Take note! Choline is commonly deficient.

Acetylcholine is made from choline, which is found in:

• Eggs • Soy • Quinoa	• Fish • Almonds • Marmite

To convert choline to acetylcholine you require:
- Vitamin C (citrus fruit, kiwi, kale, peppers, watercress, spinach, tomatoes)
- Vitamin B1 (peas, spinach, nuts, sunflower seeds, brown rice, wholegrains, red meat)

Part 2

- Vitamin B5 (nuts, seeds, sweet potato, avocado, mushrooms, yoghurt, lentils)
- Vitamin B12 (dairy, liver, eggs, beef, seafood, oily fish)

As it can be difficult to lift choline levels in the body, supplementing may be necessary. B vitamins are required for the conversion.
- 5–10g of lecithin or 1–2gm phosphatidyl choline or 300–600mg choline or 250–500mg acetyl-carnitine daily, at least one hour before eating
- 500mg vitamin C twice a day with meals
- Vitamin B Complex supplement daily, providing 25mg of all the B vitamins

2.   Be aware of your self-talk

Your self-talk is that little voice chattering away to you in your head. It's telling you things about yourself – typically how you perceive yourself and what you must/mustn't, should/shouldn't do. This internal chatter is an interference that uses up vital energy, blocks our other thinking processes and stifles creativity. We need to free ourselves from this negativity by telling ourselves it has had its say, but now it's time for it to fade away so that we can think from a different perspective.

Part
2

There is the potential for these thoughts to be self-defeating and self-sabotaging if they are too judgemental and critical. Instead of allowing you to reflect on a mistake or poor outcome and directing you to how you can improve, your self-talk generates negative attitudes about yourself and stirs up emotions that rob you of your self-esteem and self-confidence, dampen your mood and deplete your vitality and energy.

That's why it's important to be aware of just how realistic your self-talk is and what it is doing to you, and to bring in practices to control it.

Here are some tips on how to improve your self-talk:
- Praise yourself for a good job done, and hold on to the thoughts of those good things so you don't change your mind later!

- Do not let other people's inability to show appreciation affect you. Most people don't think about offering praise – they're too busy and too wrapped up in their own lives.
- Look in the mirror daily and tell yourself how fabulous you are!
- Each evening, before retiring, identify three things that have gone well that day. This is a powerful way to raise self-esteem.
- Find the good in yourself. Reflect on your strengths regularly. This knowledge will boost your self-confidence.
- Reflect on your limitations. They are not 'weaknesses' – that's a dreadful word – they're just not part of your skill set, and you have so many other things that are. There's no point in beating yourself up.
- Always have what drives you at the front of your mind. By knowing what your core values are, you will be more confident making positive decisions.
- Practise your positive self-talk frequently in your mind, or even in the mirror. This reinforces the positive – and, in time, means you will automatically think positively rather than negatively when that situation reoccurs.
- Always celebrate your successes. The reward could be something very small, such as a cup of tea, or it could be something beautiful and significant which will remind you of your achievement every time you see it.

3. Reframe the negative into the positive

A positive mindset will generate positive energy. It's as simple as that. It's about seeing the glass half-full rather than half-empty. If you look at the positive, you will trigger dopamine in the brain that will make you feel pleasure. Look at the negative, and it will trigger the stress response and send you into survival mode. You'll be fearful and anxious, which will deplete your energy and vitality. That's it.

Why is it, then, that so many of us look to the negative first? It's all about survival. What is the worst that might happen? Pre-warned is pre-armed. But in today's world the chances are that nothing is life-threatening, so being a negative thinker is a wasted attitude.

Being anxious about something, questioning your ability, is perfectly normal – but it's not if negativity dominates your thinking. Research suggests that for every one negative thought, you should have three positive thoughts.

A negative thinker attitude is a subconscious, irrational thought process where you look to the bad and discount the good. As Winston Churchill said, "The pessimist sees difficulty in every opportunity. The optimist sees the opportunity in every difficulty."

It creates a distorted version of reality, not caused by the situation itself, but by the interpretation put on it by established personal beliefs, emotions (particularly fear) and standards.

Here are some tips to become a more positive thinker:

- Make an effort to regularly check in on how you view life, people and situations. Are your views positive or negative? Spend time reviewing the negative thoughts. How much of your thinking capacity are they taking over right now? The ideal ratio should be three positive thoughts for every one negative thought.
- Break the cycle. The more you think negative thoughts, the more embedded they will become, so it is important to break this cycle. Use questions to clarify the meaning of your attitudes, to establish where you are limiting the reality, and to identify what choices you have.
- Reframe the situation. This is where you alter the event by highlighting the positive aspects. See the possibilities, not the limitations; and be solution-focused, not problem-orientated.
- Spend time with positive people. Avoid that Moaning Minnie in the office or the person who sees everything with doom and gloom – they'll drop your mood.

Part 2

- Each evening, identify three things you have to be grateful for. Maybe someone smiled at you or your report was well received. This puts you in a more positive frame of mind so eventually you begin to think more positively.
- Make your first thought at the start of each morning a positive one.
- Be calm. You need to be focused on the present (not the past or the future) and develop a clear, calm persona, which will enable you to think more positively and with greater perspective about what's going on around you.
- Take a breath. Calm the mind to engage the prefrontal cortex and use this for logical reasoning. Take three long, deep breaths, or think about something that makes you feel calm and happy – examples may be: the cat curled up by you, the children splashing in the sea or maybe a beautiful cherry tree in full blossom.
- Jot down your worries on a piece of paper and score them from 1 to 10. What can you do to reduce the score of each worry?
- Use music with an upbeat tempo during the day to energise you, and soothing music to distract your mind from the chatter and calm you in the evening.

4. Look for ways to boost your motivation and engagement

Motivation is the feeling you get when you willingly and confidently do something that needs to be done. It's about wanting to do it, whether it's because you need to (it fulfils a basic survival need), you fear looking stupid, or it excites you so you'll feel pleasure and reward.

There is little value in life and little energy generated if you carry yourself through your life on autopilot. By that I mean allowing your subconscious to lead you, with no set route or expected outcome. Not only does having a goal excite you, but your wonderful brain will also try to find ways to help you achieve that goal. Knowing what you want to achieve, and working towards it and getting success along the way, will energise you.

Your motivation may be low, though, because you fear failure and lack the confidence to move out of your comfort zone. Maybe you're not in the right frame of mind, procrastinating, or just too busy to engage into a new way of thinking. If this is the case, you'll be missing out on that spark that ignites your vitality. If you want more energy, you need to come off autopilot and take over the controls again.

Here are a few ideas on how to jump-start your motivation:

- Identify what actually motivates you. What gives you the 'oomph' to get up and get on? It's important to understand what actually does it for you. Give it some thought. It may take some time, so don't rush it. Possibilities include money, security, power, knowledge. How do these transpose into activities?
- Set yourself daily goals. What do you want to achieve? How will you achieve it, and how will you reward yourself at the end of the day?
- Set some future goals. Where would you like to be personally and professionally in 3 months, 6 months, 1 year, 5 years? What do you already have in place to get you there, and what do you need to start doing? Who can help you? How will you reward yourself when you achieve your goal?
- Be brave – try something new that will take you out of your comfort zone. Doing this will break the routine you've locked yourself into and stimulate your mind to be more active. Activity uses energy, but it returns a whole lot more.
- Make time to do the things you feel passionate about. Craft, political debating, playing sport – whatever it is. If it has been mothballed, get it out and get stuck in.
- Look at what could grow your interest and ability at work. Motivation can wane when you become stuck in a rut and bored. Maybe it's finding a new job, or studying for a qualification. Maybe changing your hours or getting involved with a project.

Part
2

Nadia's story

Nadia was finding it hard to feel any enthusiasm for her job. She would tell herself how lucky she was to have it, but that wasn't enough to engage her. Nadia told me that she had no fire, no desire and no passion for her career any more, and it was really getting her down.

She had loved her job when she first started, and was particularly pleased because she had a manager who basically left her to get on with it. She had independence and autonomy, and that was exciting. She could do the job the way she wanted to, the way she had learned to do it, using the skills and knowledge she had.

When Nadia came to see me, I felt too much autonomy was at the heart of Nadia's problem. Nadia was very capable, but she wasn't learning anything new. There was nothing to challenge her thinking. Nothing to feed her intelligence and inspire her. There were no new ways to work and no development of her capabilities.

Being too autonomous meant Nadia's competence had stagnated. She was bored, and boredom leaves you dissatisfied and robs you of energy. If Nadia wanted to feel energised by her career again, she needed to find ways that would grow her capabilities and interest in her work again. Only she could do this.

With some coaching, Nadia prepared for a conversation with her manager. She asked if she could work with him (note **with** him) on a project that would grow a new skill set. She had some ideas she could put to him. She also looked at studying part-time for a master's degree, and prepared a proposal for her employer to fund this.

As Nadia saw the results, she realised that she had taken the opportunity to work autonomously too far. A career is a continuous process of learning and developing new skills and knowledge, and the only way to remain engaged and motivated by work (and energised) is to find opportunities to grow your interest.

5. Be grateful

> *"Cultivate the habit of being grateful for every good thing that comes to you, and to give thanks continuously. And because all things have contributed to your advancement, you should include all things in your gratitude."*

Ralph Waldo Emerson

It's not money that makes you happy, but gratitude – and if you're happy, you're more likely to feel energised.

Gratitude is about being thankful and able to show appreciation for what you have, and for things others have done for you. Gratitude generates positive emotions, triggers dopamine in the brain and energises you.

Here are some ways to cultivate gratitude:

- Keep a gratitude diary. Before you settle down to sleep, record three things in your diary you are grateful for that day. This helps your mind to feel more positive about your day and reduces elevated stress hormones.
- Be generous to others. The gratitude they show you will give you a boost.
- Pay someone a compliment. Make sure it's genuine, and if a compliment is returned, accept it willingly.
- Always show your appreciation for something someone does for you. A small note, email or call, or include it in a conversation.
- Volunteer. Being kind to someone stimulates dopamine and serotonin, two chemicals in the brain associated with feeling good. Being kind to others provides a sense of reward and happiness which you may be struggling to get at work.
- Be spontaneously kind to someone. Get them a coffee when you're making yours, or lend a quick hand if you see they're under time pressure.

6.   Laugh more every day

As the saying goes, "Laughter is the best medicine." And it's true. Laughter is a healer. It increases blood flow to the brain, making you more alert. It reduces sympathetic nervous system activity, switching you to the more relaxed parasympathetic nervous system, and, in so doing, reduces stress hormones and eases anxiety and tension. It strengthens immunity again and increases endorphins – the feel-good hormones. Laughter boosts mental wellbeing, and all in all it's absolutely fabulous!

Laughter grabs your attention. It's amazing how the mind will recognise it and put you on alert. When you hear it, you will be tempted to stop what you're doing and find out what's so funny. Was it a joke, or reliving a funny situation? Your curiosity will be fired up – and with this your energy!

You can bring more laughter into your life by smiling.

- Spend time with happy, jovial people who have a good sense of humour.
- Watch a funny movie or TV show.
- Try out a laughter yoga class.
- Laugh at yourself – self-deprecating humour can really lighten conversations.
- Don't take life too seriously. Make time for the lighter side of life, such as enjoying the company of family and friends.
- Burst into song – the shock will make others laugh, then you will!
- Make dress-down Friday a dressing-up day.
- Subscribe to daily email jokes.
- Take time out regularly to close your eyes and smile.

7.   Don't be afraid to ask for help

When life becomes too much, don't be afraid to ask for help. It is not a sign of weakness – in fact I would put it as a sign of strength.

You want to feel better, but you know you can't make it happen on your own.

Talk to someone close to you – a family member or friend. This is someone who you know you can confidently share your challenges with. It could be that they have already approached you and you've dismissed their offer of help, but it's never too late.

Better still, talk to your manager. But if your manager is the problem, speak to HR or occupational health, or utilise your company's Employee Assistance Programme counselling contract if they have one. It's a free confidential service that allows you to talk about anything from financial worries to childcare issues as well as stress-related problems.

If you need it, take time out. A day each side of the weekend may be enough, but if not, take a complete break, with no work interruptions. Maybe your employer offers sabbaticals if you have been there for a certain period of time. These may require a discussion with your manager, HR or occupational health. It is becoming a more common occurrence, so don't feel embarrassed, ashamed or cross with yourself. You have not failed – it's because you have done so much that you're in this situation. Turn your life around and use your experience to learn, change and grow.

Part 2

Activities to learn more about how far positivity optimises your energy

Activity 1: Signs and symptoms of neurotransmitter deficiency

1. Tick or highlight the signs and symptoms in the next table that are currently relevant to you.

Dopamine	Serotonin
I have trouble waking in the morning	I am anxious or 'on edge'
I need a caffeine drink to get going	I worry more than I used to
I have little interest in activities and hobbies	I am depressed
I lack drive and enthusiasm	I am worse in the dark winter months
I struggle to get going and finish tasks	I have trouble falling asleep and wake often
I feel bored and apathetic	I struggle with the same thoughts going over and over in my head
I feel depressed	I obsess that things are right
I lack focus and concentration	I can quickly change my mood
I am less creative than usual	I can be irritable or angry, or go into a rage
I find it difficult to take in details	I respond poorly to stressful situations
I am easily fatigued	I get frequent headaches or migraines
I crave stimulants (eg, alcohol, caffeine, nicotine, drugs)	I am very self-critical and have low self-confidence and self-esteem
I have little interest in sex and love	I have digestive problems such as constipation
I find it hard to handle stressful situations	I crave sweet foods
I have restless leg syndrome	I have a low pain threshold
Gamma-Aminobutyric Acid (GABA)	Acetylcholine
I feel anxious and agitated	I forget common things I should know
I suffer panic attacks	I suffer from 'brain fog' and have difficulty concentrating
I find it difficult to focus	I have trouble following what people say

Part
2

I have trouble relaxing and chilling out	I have trouble recalling what I have just read
I feel overwhelmed	I find it difficult to find the right word
I have racing thoughts	I find it too much to socialise
I feel stiff, tense and uneasy	I feel overwhelmed
I have a tendency to shake and twitch	I feel disorientated
I feel nervous	I easily feel tired
I have heart palpitations or feel short of breath	I struggle with muscle aches and weakness
I have a nervous tummy (butterflies)	I struggle to do mental maths or work things out in my head
I need alcohol to relax	I lose the train of my thought when speaking
I am sensitive to bright light and loud noise	I misplace things and forget where I've put them
I have trouble getting to sleep	I have dry eyes
I struggle with stressful situations	I have lost my creativity

Part
2

2. If you mostly agree with these statements, it is likely that that particular neurotransmitter is deficient and requires some support. Turn to pages 196–199 for suggestions on how to make improvements.

A urine test can also confirm your neurotransmitter status. *See www.susanscott.co.uk* for further details.

Activity 2: My best manager

Think about the person who has been the best manager you have ever had.

1. What words describe that person? Record your ideas below.

2. When you have exhausted your ideas, tick the words that best describe your positive feelings (positive emotions).

3. When you think about this person, how does it make you feel? Identifying this will identify positive emotions that energise you.

A powerful way to fuel positivity is by doing or saying something that makes someone else feel good, or doing or saying something that makes you feel good. Try to incorporate this into your everyday life. Eventually it will switch off the negative chatter in your head and help you see the positive side of life.

Activity 3: Positive-thinking activities
Here are some ideas to get you started. Highlight or tick the activity below that you will do to create a positive mindset:

Activity	✓
During a conversation with someone, I will ask what I can do for them. Note, this is not about what *they* can do for *you*, so do not request it.	
Each day I will praise one person.	
Each day I will praise myself for something I did well.	
Each week I will do an unexpected favour for someone.	
Each day I will express my appreciation to someone, either by personal note or face to face.	
I will smile and say "hi" to everyone who comes within two metres of me.	
I will always focus on what I can do, not on what I can't do.	
I will always focus on what went well, not what went badly.	
I will argue with my inner critic. I am good, I am worthy. Practise in the mirror!	
I will give myself permission to make a mistake – after all, I am human. If I make a mistake, I'll acknowledge it, learn from it, then mentally walk away from it.	

Part
2

The 7 steps to optimum energy

Activity	✓
Each day I will count my blessings – the things I have which I am grateful for.	
Each month I will offer some time to help a local charity.	
I will put a red sticker on my watch. Whenever I look at my watch, it will alert me to stop what I'm doing, take three deep breaths, then reflect on something positive.	
I will use humour and make people smile or laugh.	
I will spend the first five minutes in any new activity being positive and cheerful.	

Positivity can also come from feeling good about ourselves. We are all special in our own way and have a unique array of characteristics that make us so. Typically, we spend little time thinking about what makes us special – our personal brand. But this knowledge can boost our energy and motivation, particularly when we're low on energy and feeling down.

Part 2

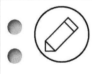

Activity 4: The 'Big-I'

1. Give some thought to what makes you special. It might be that you're good at finishing things, or maybe you notice detail, or perhaps you willingly give your time to people.
2. Take a piece of plain paper, and, using different-coloured pens, record your ideas. Start each idea with "I am...". For example, "I am always cheerful", "I am calm in a crisis".
3. Photocopy your page and put it somewhere where you will regularly see it: maybe on the back of your wardrobe door, or inside the front cover of your diary. Regularly reflect on it, particularly if your positivity or energy is being challenged.

Gratitude is an affirmation of the good things happening in our lives, around us and around the world. Thinking about what we have to be grateful for is a powerful way to become more positive and optimistic, and has been shown to create more vitality and happiness.

Activity 5: Gratitude diary

1. Use a special notebook and dedicate it to recording all the things you can be grateful for.

2. Each evening, before you go to sleep, record three things that you are grateful for that day. There may have been events that occurred during the day that instantly come to mind.

   When you've had a bad day, thinking of things can be more difficult. On these occasions, look to the very simple things around you: nature; someone or something that has made you smile; having a friend, relative or pet; or even the weather!

3. If you are experiencing a tough day, look back over your book. Pick out one gratitude point and focus on it for a few moments. Consider why you are grateful for it. Visualise this in your mind and tune in to your senses. How does it make you feel? Hopefully this will calm you, create a positive state and energise you.

Life is beset with problems, and although we can often go with the flow, at other times these problems can really pull us down. Hindsight is a wonderful thing, so the voice in our head repeatedly churns over what we should have done to avoid it. That's good for learning for next time, but this internal chatter by our inner critic can sap energy.

We have to tell ourselves this chatter is normal, then try to move on before it totally consumes us.

Use this exercise to get your thoughts down on paper and get the situation into perspective. The aim is to help you look on the bright side of the situation: what did actually go well, what you could learn from it for the future.

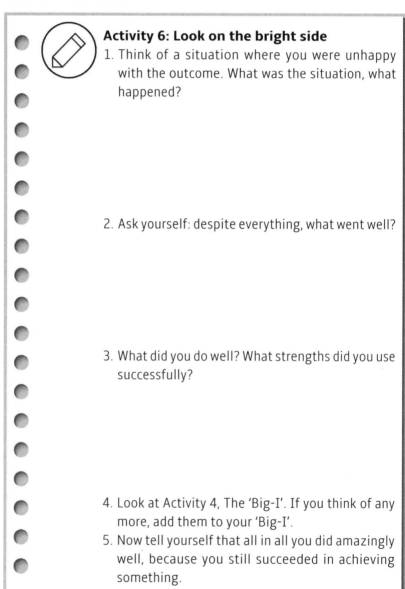

Activity 6: Look on the bright side

1. Think of a situation where you were unhappy with the outcome. What was the situation, what happened?

2. Ask yourself: despite everything, what went well?

3. What did you do well? What strengths did you use successfully?

4. Look at Activity 4, The 'Big-I'. If you think of any more, add them to your 'Big-I'.

5. Now tell yourself that all in all you did amazingly well, because you still succeeded in achieving something.

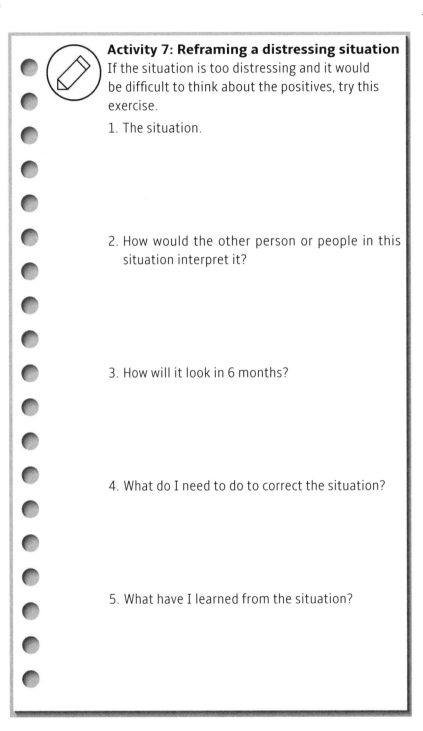

Activity 7: Reframing a distressing situation

If the situation is too distressing and it would be difficult to think about the positives, try this exercise.

1. The situation.

2. How would the other person or people in this situation interpret it?

3. How will it look in 6 months?

4. What do I need to do to correct the situation?

5. What have I learned from the situation?

Part
2

Your reflections

What has resonated with you while reading Step 7: Positivity for optimum energy?

- What have you learned about yourself?
- What have you learned about how positivity affects the state of your energy?
- What do you need to start doing that you have not done before?
- What other thoughts do you have?

Part 2

CHAPTER 11

50 ways to optimise your energy

For each of the steps to optimising your personal energy contained in this book, I have explained seven ways in which you could improve that element.

If you are feeling tired all the time and want to break away and boost your energy, here is a summary of them all, plus one extra. You may spend so much time giving to others that it leaves very little capacity for you. If you want to begin the journey of boosting your energy and genuinely experience the benefits, you need to be kind to yourself. Keep this at the forefront of your mind: it will help you to prioritise your recovery.

1. Feed your mitochondria
2. Balance your blood sugar
3. Reduce your stimulant intake
4. Stay well hydrated
5. Nurture your thyroid gland
6. Boost your microbiome
7. Monitor how you eat when feeling stressed
8. Create a bedtime routine

9. Make your bedroom sleep-friendly
10. Eat right to sleep well
11. Banish worry and anxiety
12. Take control of your technology
13. Follow practices to calm your mind
14. Get a dose of morning sunlight
15. Practise deep breathing
16. Don't just sit there, do something!
17. Get up and walk more!
18. Bring movement into your work life
19. Power up your home routine
20. Find an activity that boosts your oxygen intake
21. Use technology to track your movement
22. Mix with high-energy, positive people
23. Find more opportunities to socialise

Part 2

24. Schedule social events in your diary
25. Develop your empathy skills
26. Deal with difficult people
27. Get out and network
28. Give people your attention
29. Know who you are
30. Identify what's important to you
31. Live according to your values
32. Have a clear vision of where you want your life to go
33. Do something every day you're passionate about
34. Be curious
35. Recognise what brings you joy
36. Know how you spend your time
37. Plan how you will use your time
38. Take back control of digital technology
39. Learn to say no
40. Keep a stress log

41. Work in 60-minute cycles
42. Schedule in recovery time
43. Boost your brain's chemical messengers
44. Be aware of your self-talk
45. Reframe the negative into the positive
46. Look for ways to boost your motivation and engagement
47. Be grateful
48. Laugh more every day
49. Don't be too afraid to ask for help
50. Be kind to yourself

Part
2

Part 2

PART 3

Your 7 Steps to Optimum Energy plan

CHAPTER 12

Your action plan to optimise your energy

There is a Chinese proverb that tells us, "He that is afraid to shake the dice will never throw a six." Being low on energy plays havoc with your confidence and self-worth and makes you fearful of what else could happen to you. It's natural. I can remember the times when I have suffered from low energy – just how fearful I was of doing anything that would put the tiny bit of capacity to function I had at risk. My youngest child woke every night for three years. It took me years to switch off the voice in my head telling me I must get to bed early to conserve my energy. But I now know, if you don't move to action, you won't build your energy. It's as simple as that. No pain, no gain. If you want more energy, you have to do something new.

This book contains an enormous amount of information to get you thinking about your life and the changes that can make a difference to your energy.

Be aware, though, you cannot do everything at once. If you try to, you will be overwhelmed and fail, leaving you demotivated and in a worse state than before. Instead, take small steps, choosing activities that you are more likely to stick to and that will have the greatest impact. These may be making better food choices to balance your blood sugar, or improving your sleep hygiene and incorporating rest periods into your day. Stay committed to doing these activities until they become a habit: the more you do an activity, the easier it will become, particularly when you notice a difference in your energy. Once it has become a habit, you can add another activity, and so it goes on. This is a process that takes time and for which there is no quick-fix pill. You have to take control, but you must pace yourself.

Begin the process by picking out anything that caught your attention: your light bulb moments. Go back through the book and review each section. How would you summarise the book?

My light bulb moments

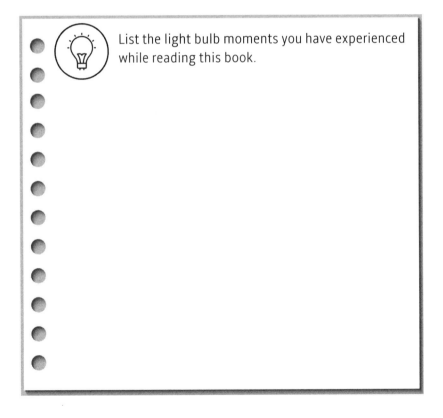

List the light bulb moments you have experienced while reading this book.

Part

3

My energy improvement chart – the way forward

Now look in detail at how you scored on each exercise within the book.

1. Score how you performed in the exercises in each section in the following way:
   - E: Excellent
   - R: Room for improvement
   - A: Attention required
   - U: Urgent action required

2. Identify what action you will take. Review the book, particularly the seven 'energy-boosting' ways outlined in each chapter and any lists of tips included, for ideas.

Chapter	Score	What did you learn from this section?	Action required to improve your score
What is energy?			
The energy zappers			
Step 1: Nutrition for optimum energy			
Step 2: Sleep for optimum energy			

Step 3: Movement for optimum energy			
Step 4: Connectivity for optimum energy			
Step 5: Purpose for optimum energy			
Step 6: Balance for optimum energy			
Step 7: Positivity for optimum energy			

Part 3

Tracking your progress

It is important to regularly track how your energy is improving and whether you need to make any further changes to your diet and lifestyle.

1. Use the chart on the next pages to score yourself on a scale of 1 to 10 according to how full of energy and vitality you are, where 10 = full of energy and vitality and 1 = running on empty.
2. Consider why you have given yourself this score: how are you physically, mentally and emotionally?
3. What new rituals can you develop to raise your score to a new, higher level?

Your 7 Steps to Optimum Energy plan

Part 3

At the start of the programme	My score: 1–10:
Why this score:	
Further rituals:	

After 30 days of action	My score: 1–10:
Why this score:	
Further rituals:	

After 60 days of action	My score: 1–10:

Why this score:

Further rituals:

After 90 days of action	My score: 1–10:

Why this score:

Further rituals:

Part
3

It is very easy to come up with great ideas about what you need to do to optimise your energy while you're reading this book. You may even maintain this enthusiasm for a time afterwards, but once you're out in the real world there's a great danger of returning to your old habits – it's much easier!

New habits take effort, time and lots of practice. Some days will prove difficult, but that doesn't mean you give up if you've gone off course one day. Just start again the next day.

You are much more likely to continue if you are able to reinforce the benefits you are experiencing. Here are a few suggestions to help you.

- Keep a diary of your progress. Use a notebook diary specifically for this purpose. Record one thing each day that takes you a step towards feeling fully energised. Consider what happened that day, what you learned, what surprised you and the outcome. Regularly review it.

- Write regular letters or emails to yourself capturing what you did and how it made you feel, physically, mentally and emotionally. Keep these emails stored in an Energy folder.

- Use Instagram, and each day take a photo that captures what you did to boost your energy. It could be a photo of a healthy lunch choice, a picture of the park at lunchtime, a hug with your child when you got home – whatever inspires you. Regularly look back over these and wallow in the wonderful feeling it gives you.

CHAPTER 13

Your journey to optimum energy

My aim when writing this book was that, through my professional learning and personal experience, I could help others recover from feeling fatigued, regain their lost energy and get their life back, just as I have managed to do so.

As you have hopefully realised by reading my book, there are many ways to achieve optimum energy, and you certainly don't have to live a life locked in to a state of exhaustion – it just takes some tweaks to your diet, your lifestyle and your mental attitude, and the potential to be bubbling with enthusiasm and vitality again is there.

You've read the theory, engaged with the life stories and hopefully picked up some valuable tips – so the time has come to start your journey. Energy is your birthright; it's the basic currency of life, but it is not a given. Today's highly pressured life, filled with energy zappers, requires you to proactively manage your energy. Things will not get better on their own. It requires thought and investment. You must take personal responsibility, and only you alone can make it happen. Sadly there is no sachet of magic fairy dust that comes free with this book to save you the effort (how I wish I had that myself at times). You have to decide what is within your power to do, and move to action.

I've covered a lot in this book, so it is important to prioritise your actions. You need to be realistic and not take on too many things, nor try to do too much. It's of no help to you if you're having to force yourself through gritted teeth to do something, because the inevitable "What's the point?" will raise its head, and you'll only give up.

None of my tips are too onerous, but if you are struggling with low energy, you will need to be selective when choosing what to take on board. There's no way you could do everything I've suggested. There's a chance that you're doing some of my suggestions already, and there's every chance that some may be beyond your capability at this time – but the important thing is to start with what inspires you the most.

Start with the easiest suggestion that will give you the most benefit. Focus on one or two areas to improve. It might be a question of making some simple swaps or adding a new, healthier routine into your life. Look at your responses to the Energy Risk Factors Questionnaire in Chapter 3 to determine where you should focus your actions. Once you have embedded these into your lifestyle, look at two more areas, get them going and build up gradually. It could be that you want to improve your diet, so eating more protein at each meal as a way to balance your blood sugar is more achievable initially than reducing your coffee intake – this can come at a later time. Or incorporating a morning walk as part of your morning commute will make you feel stronger and more confident before you can sign up for a gym membership.

Pace yourself. To feel measurable improvements in your energy, you need to take your journey at a pace that you can manage, where you build your energy gradually. This means a pace that is not so taxing that it exhausts, overwhelms or demotivates you so you give up – or, worst of all, that it robs you of the little energy you do have.

Trust me. My professional experience as a psychologist and nutritional therapist tells me that you will achieve greater success if you take small, steady steps where you make gradual changes which become embedded as good habits and routines. 'Gently does it' is much better for you than 'going for it, all guns blazing'. Do that and you run the risk of burning yourself out. A step-by-step approach also provides you with the opportunity to discover what the true underlying causes of your low energy may be – and, as a result, what the most powerful and pertinent techniques may be for you. This is particularly important to know should your energy happen to drop back again in the future.

When I was struggling with low energy, I didn't have the capacity to think straight and remember what I was supposed to do to get me out of this place of fatigue at times. To help me, I found that if I scheduled my new activities in my diary, I had a central place to coordinate my journey from. This helped me to make my actions habit-forming. These activities were still appointments, but they were appointments with myself, and my diary became my road map for my journey to better health and energy.

As your energy increases, you may find it comes in small bursts, where your energy improves, then plateaus; then you try something else and it improves again, then plateaus again. This is perfectly normal. Optimising your energy is a journey, and it's quite typical to have stops and starts along the way and for some of you to find it easier than others.

Maintaining your personal energy is an ongoing activity, and returning from a place of fatigue takes time. If you're not feeling it, don't worry: the time will come when you will, so have faith. I've had two experiences when I've woken up one day and thought, "Hello, welcome back" – but before these happened, I had my doubts that I would ever feel the real energised me again.

This means *hang in there*. What you don't want is for your good intentions to slip away. You're likely to feel enthusiastic at the beginning of your journey, but sustaining it is a whole different ball game, particularly when all those challenges in life are still there.

Part
3

Should you get those moments when your motivation starts to wane, you then need to find a way to fire up your enthusiasm again. When some of my clients have reached this point, they have found it incredibly helpful to do a bit of visualisation, imagining what a life of bountiful energy could feel like. It's no different from an athlete imagining themselves winning their race and being on top of the podium. Visualisation puts you back in control of your life again.

There is the possibility that you will not realise just how far you've come on your journey. I can be a bit like that. I'm not one for dwelling on the past – which is a good thing – but it does mean I forget how bad I may have felt. Whether this is you or not, I always recommend that, at the start of your journey, you score yourself out of 10 for how much energy you have, where 10 is high. Whenever your motivation starts to wane, score yourself again. For example, if you started at a score of 3 but now have a score of 4, you've made a fantastic improvement. Give some thought to what you could do now to get to a score of 5. Don't even countenance getting to 9 or 10 at this stage – it's woefully unrealistic – but 5 will be a great step in the right direction.

If your motivation does wane, try imagining yourself in a future where you have all the energy you require. Make a mental list of all the good things you're going to be able to do with your new-found energy. How would this make you feel? What effect would this have on your family, friends and colleagues?

If you're going to find it hard to keep hold of these thoughts, write them down and regularly remind yourself why you're on this journey. If you place copies of your written thoughts in key places around your house and workplace, you can regularly refresh yourself on the upside of making so much effort. To complement this, by keeping these thoughts at the forefront of your mind, your mind will look for opportunities to help you achieve success.

I cannot predict exactly what form your renewed energy will take

– physical, mental or both. Healing your body takes time and, yes, energy. What I do know is that if you stick at it, you'll reap the benefits. By being brave, determined and positive, you have a greater chance of turning your life around and boosting your Life Force. This is the pathway to something better which will stand you in good stead for the rest of your life. You can do it.

The point to remember is that any improvement is a gift, and an asset to you and your life. Be patient. Gradually, you will feel a difference. A few small embers may be enough to reignite the fire, or those few embers may be like a pilot light waiting for fuel to ignite – meaning you have to try something else as well. Or maybe you start something and have to make your own personal adjustments.

I'm not able to predict how long your journey will take. It depends on the underlying causes of your low energy, so it cannot be predicted. No matter how long it is, I want you to know that you are not alone. I feel so passionate about the power of optimum energy, I want you to know that I am here to help you to continue along your journey.

With such a vast and interesting topic, I could have written an encyclopaedia. There is only so much room for explanation in a book. The suggestions in this book are the most powerful. If you are looking for further insights and ideas, check out some of the tips leaflets on a variety of topics which you can download at *www.susanscott.co.uk*. There's also a newsletter you can sign up for. If you're a user of social media, I also regularly post tips and explanations on Instagram and Twitter as @The_Energy_Aunt.

There are many paths to healing, and with every bit of research I also learn more. What really brings everything alive for me is people's experiences. We are all unique individuals, and so there is no magic bullet or one-size-fits-all approach. Let me know how you get on: your stories of transformation are always of great interest to me. It's real people that bring this topic alive, and I for one am still learning. You can contact me on *energy@susanscott.co.uk*.

Part
3

I feel so privileged that you have taken me into your life. My wish for you is that my book will be a supportive companion for you on your journey to optimum energy. As The Buddha so profoundly said, "No matter how hard the past, you can always begin again." You don't have to live your life devoid of energy and vitality. Start over again: today is a new day.

Yours in health and Bon Voyage!

I wish you a safe and successful journey.

Susan

Part
3

An invitation to connect and engage

Keywords: Nutrition, Energy, Optimum Energy, Healing, Adrenals, Thyroid, Drainers, Balance, Positivity, Sleep, Wellbeing, Restore, Tranquillity, Personal Development, Mindfulness, Motivational, Empowerment, Life Force, Transformational, Struggling, Tired, Tiredness, Exhausted, Fatigue, Brain fog, Energised, Vitality, Mood, Concentration, Water, Food, Diet, Mindset, Health, Fitness, Mental health, Revolutionary.

Digitally connect: I'm passionate about engaging and connecting with people. Here are the ways in which we can keep in touch and share your journeys of transformation. Remember, I know what I'm talking about. I'm a scientist with a master's degree, and I've lived long enough and have the professional expertise to cut right through the fads and the opinions of the unqualified.

Instagram and Twitter: @The_Energy_Aunt "Tips from an expert on how to boost energy & prevent burnout. Psychologist – Registered Nutritionist MBANT – Best-selling author"

Website: *www.susanscott.co.uk* for tips on a variety of topics and my blog.

Email: contact me on *energy@susanscott.co.uk*.

For high-value speaking engagements and workshops: I am passionate about people's wellbeing and success. I believe wholeheartedly that it is within everyone's power to live their life with energy and vitality: they just need to know how and be motivated to make the necessary changes a lifelong practice. My speaker events are designed to inspire people to take ownership. I apply my extensive academic, real-life and work experiences to energise and engage people as I share my insights and advice. Combining my passion for the topic with a powerful and empowering speaking style, I bring topics to life by interacting extensively with my audience and guiding them through practical exercises, leaving them ready to act and flourish. Topics include career resilience, personal resilience, preventing burnout, career development, building personal energy, and thyroid and adrenal health.

News and press: I'm always willing to comment on news topics relating to energy, burnout and career resilience, answer your questions, or provide tips and quotes for publication. Contact my publicist, Helen Lewis, at *helenlewis@literallypr.com*.

Gratitude

I will be eternally grateful to the many people who have touched my life and played their part in optimising my energy and vitality. A heartfelt thanks to you all, because I now feel ready to share what I have learnt with the world.

I would never have had the energy to write this book without my wonderful husband, John, who has been there with me the whole way along my career journey. You understand me and believe in me and my message, and have been a never-ending source of encouragement, particularly when I doubt myself. Your unconditional love, support, shared creativity and, without question, all those healthy meals you cooked that kept me going, made the writing possible, even enjoyable. You are my rock.

My wonderful family. My beautiful daughters, Lucy and Ysabel, and vivacious son-in-law, Dean, who have been so patient with me as I've rabbited on about my book ideas and forced manuscripts on you to read and critique. You have helped me to understand who I am and bring so much joy to my life. My beautiful sister, Jaki, who is always there for me. You nurtured me as my thyroid packed up and I spiralled into the depths of despair. You gave me the strength and collateral to fight the medical profession for a diagnosis until I finally met the brilliant consultant endocrinologist Professor David

Russell-Jones and I found my life again. My mother, who was always such a bundle of energy, who lit up every room she entered.

I dread to think where my energy would be without my special friends. My friends who share my passion for walking, dancing, food and the arts – you bring so much fun and laughter into my life. My school friends Jane Clarke, Jenny Spivey and Julia Sanghani, who I've known for ever and feel so at ease with. You are my personal psychotherapists who put me right with your pearls of wisdom. I would go to the end of the earth and back for you. Dr Rachel Nicoll, who referred me onto a toxic metal research programme: I will be forever grateful.

My incredible dance teachers, Kate Shaw and Steve and Charlotte King, who boost my energy through movement and a hell of a lot of laughter. My yoga teachers, Julie Gibson and Lee Hopkins, whose spiritual insights have touched my life so much and calm my chaotic mind. Your advice and wisdom are diffused throughout this book.

I am so grateful to the countless people who have helped to get this book from a few scrappy chapters to what it is now. My supercharged, insightful, talented publicist and agent, Helen Lewis of The Literally Agency. For your belief in me and that this book needed to be out there. For your tenacity, and for helping me along my journey. You are awesome and it's such a pleasure working with you.

For Tracey Dobby and the dream team at Eclipse Publishing and Media. Tracey, who gets my message and wants to share it with the world: that means so much to me. Graham Hughes from GH Editorial and Margaret Hunter from Daisy Editorial for your skilful copy-editing and design, and Aimee Coveney for the high-energy cover design. Thank you from the bottom of my heart for believing in me. I am eternally grateful that my book landed with you.

Over my career, there are so many people I have learned from and am still learning from. I will always be so grateful to everyone I have come into contact with from around the world, both professionally and personally. To the people I have met on my workshops, in my clinics and at speaking events. Your stories and insights have given my knowledge depth and meaning, and have inspired me to share what I know through the written word now. Thank you for listening to me and allowing me to be part of your journey to health and success. I am particularly grateful to everyone who has allowed me to share their story in this book.

I thank my professional colleagues who I have worked alongside. A particular debt of gratitude goes to my business partners, Dr Derek Mowbray and Barbara Leigh at The Resilience Training Company, who encouraged me to write a small guide to optimising personal energy three years ago. It seemed inconceivable at the time that these few words would provide the framework for this manuscript. So much inspiration comes from our business meetings as we humorously bounce ideas, models and theories back and forth. Thank you.

My very talented friend Anne Perret, who I've spent many an hour discussing thyroid disease and adrenal health with. You so generously reviewed my original small guide to personal energy and gave me the confidence to publish. You are a very special person.

My work is evidence-based, and I feel indebted to all the scientists, doctors and researchers who feed my hunger for knowledge and practical application with their research and analysis. I'd also like to thank Patrick Holford and Jeff Bland PhD for inspiring me to study nutrition and functional medicine, which created my mind-body specialism.

About Susan Scott

MSc, FCIPD, FISMA, MABP, MBANT

Susan is a business psychologist, a registered nutritional therapist, a trainer, a consultant and a coach, as well as a public speaker and an Amazon best-selling author.

She has worked extensively in the information technology, management consultancy, finance, legal and charity sectors, and has designed and delivered major change management projects and management, leadership and wellbeing programmes for numerous private and public sector organisations across the UK, Europe, the USA and Australasia. In tandem with consulting work, Susan ran a nutritional therapy clinic for executives experiencing burnout.

Susan brings a blended mind-and-body approach to her work. She believes passionately that everyone deserves to work in ways that foster their resilience, performance and career. And, because of her extensive experience in working within organisations, she is very aware of the drive and passion that people bring to their work, and why this needs to be managed in ways that optimise their energy.

Susan has an MSc in Organisational Behaviour from the University of London and a Diploma in Nutritional Therapy (Distinction) from the Institute for Optimum Nutrition, and is registered with the Nutritional Therapy Council.

She is a Fellow of the Chartered Institute of Personnel and Development and a Fellow of the International Stress Management Association. She is also a Principal Member of the Association for Business Psychology and a Member of the British Association of Applied Nutrition and Nutritional Therapy.

She is a past chair of the trustees of the International Stress Management Association (ISMA^UK), is the author of *How to Have an Outstanding Career* and *How to Prevent Burnout* and is the co-author of *The Manager's Role in Stress Prevention* with Dr Derek Mowbray.

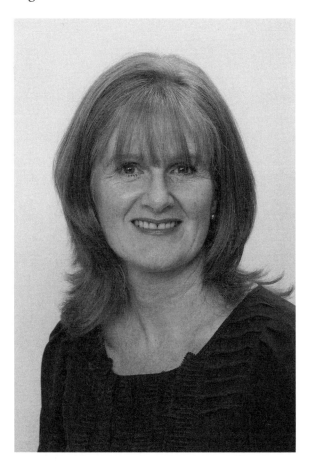

My energy notes

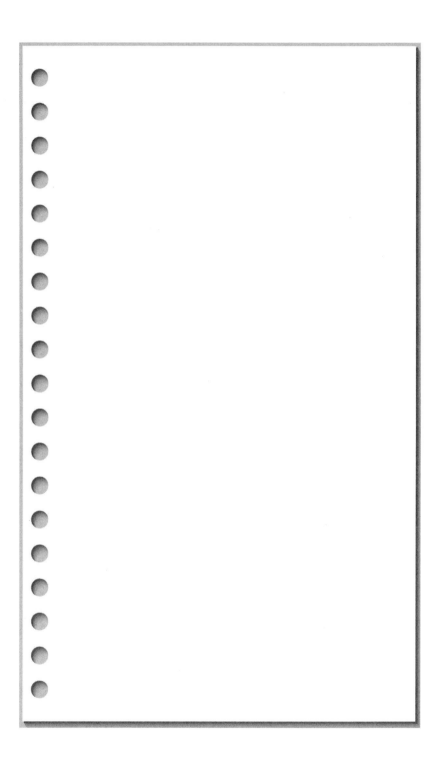